MEND OR MOVE ON

MEMO OR MOVE ON

Mend

or

Move On

A GUIDE TO HEALING OR LEAVING TOXIC RELATIONSHIPS

Kate King, MA, LPC, ATR-BC

JOHNS HOPKINS UNIVERSITY PRESS

Baltimore

© 2026 Johns Hopkins University Press
All rights reserved. Published 2026
Printed in the United States of America on acid-free paper
9 8 7 6 5 4 3 2 1

Johns Hopkins University Press
2715 North Charles Street
Baltimore, Maryland 21218
www.press.jhu.edu

Library of Congress Cataloging-in-Publication Data is available.

A catalog record for this book is available from the British Library.

ISBN 978-1-4214-5347-7 (hardcover)
ISBN 978-1-4214-5348-4 (paperback)
ISBN 978-1-4214-5349-1 (ebook)

*Special discounts are available for bulk purchases of this book. For more
information, please contact Special Sales at specialsales@jh.edu.*

EU GPSR Authorized Representative
LOGOS EUROPE, 9 rue Nicolas Poussin,
17000, La Rochelle, France
E-mail: Contact@logoseurope.eu

This work is for my Core4.
Danny, Bridger, and Heidi,
thank you for helping me learn every day
what healthy love looks and feels like.
I am endlessly grateful for each of you.

Contents

Author's Note

The intention of this book is to provide helpful information on the subjects discussed. It is not intended to be used for the diagnosis or treatment of any specific medical, psychiatric, or mental health issues. Please always consult with your primary health provider if you feel uncertain about decisions that could affect your health. If you feel emotionally unstable and at risk of harming yourself or someone else, please immediately call 911 or go to your nearest emergency room.

All names and identifying information of the people portrayed in case studies included in this book have been changed to maintain confidentiality.

Definitions

Toxic

The Oxford English Dictionary*'s definition:* "Poisonous; harmful or dangerous to health or life."[1]

Toxic Person

Kate's definition: A person who preys on others to satisfy their dysfunctional need for control, power, or security. They use strategies like shame, manipulation, or coercion to meet their own needs at the expense of another. Toxic people often operate from profoundly unhealed trauma and/or mental illness. They are inclined toward vindictive ends in order to avoid the healing that could free them from their poisonous relational tendencies. They can profoundly harm the mind, heart, body, or spirit of another in their insatiable quest to achieve superiority and control.

Toxic Relationship

Kate's definition: A connection between individuals that promotes disease, unwellness, and/or trauma due to its harmful qualities to the mind, body, heart, or soul. Participants may be toxic in their behaviors, personalities, or qualities, or the dynamic itself may have become toxic without necessitating toxicity in personalities of the participants themselves outside of the bond.

Healthy Relationship

Kate's definition: A connection between individuals that promotes health, well-being, genuine connection, and belonging due to supportive qualities that nourish the mind, body, heart, and soul. Participants feel safe and valued in the dynamic, which leads to growth and vitality in the experiences of all involved.

---

1. *Oxford English Dictionary* (online), under "toxic, adj. & n." https://www.oed.com/search/dictionary/?scope=Entries&q=toxic.

MEND OR MOVE ON

Introduction

Life Is Too Short for Harmful Relationships

Human beings were not given claws or fur or razor-sharp teeth for survival. We were given our big brains, opposable thumbs, and one another. Although community and relationships play a monumental role in the safety, survival, well-being, and productivity of humankind, our interpersonal dynamics also seem to cause universal pain and suffering. That relationships are exclusively joy-filled and easy is an illusion we all must face—some people earlier than others. To reduce the experience of our relational dances to an expectation of simple joy is akin to making a sphere one-dimensional. It only renders flat the wholeness and brilliance of our capacity for connectivity.

If you're a human being, you have relationships. If you're reading this book, you care about those connections and want them to flourish. When I speak of "relationships," I mean more than your romantic partnership. Many people go astray when they identify their significant other as the only relationship in their life that requires intentional tending. This book applies to each and every one of your complex, meaningful, layered, and messy relationships: your friends, colleagues and clients, children, neighbors, acquaintances, intimate and extended family members—even your dentist and hairdresser. Every person who has a role in your life is on the other end of a tether that binds the two of you in your relational dynamic. Whether you know it or admit it, each connection requires varying degrees of intention and thoughtfulness to maintain healthfully—if it should be maintained at all.

In my nearly two decades of clinical work as a licensed professional counselor and board-certified art therapist, relationships have arisen, hands down, as the most common client complaint and symptomology of unhappiness. I have also lived this reality throughout the decades of my life in many forms of personal experience. I am familiar with the rocky terrain of knowing in my gut that cutting ties is the only way to remain healthy and safe because I have made the infinitely challenging decision to estrange myself from abusive family members. I have also ended misaligned friendships and professional relationships for the purpose of choosing my integrity and well-being instead of collapsing into the peacekeeping and compliance those connections required.

One such relationship rift happened over this very book you are reading. After being asked to replace the hope and light of my work with a loud, controversial perspective that condones taking a machete to all imperfect relationships, I stepped away from a powerful professional connection that may have opened many doors for me. The price would have been my authenticity, and that price was simply too high. A Post-it note on my desk continues to remind me: "If it costs my peace, it's too expensive." On the flip side, I have also repaired relationships that were in a downward freefall, working together with my counterpart in those dynamics to salvage a bond that we both agreed was worth keeping. So, you see, it is not one-size-fits-all. Most important things in life aren't.

The decision point between staying in or leaving a misaligned relationship is a potent one that certainly falls into the "relationship issues" category for many people. The knife edge of discerning when to stay and when to leave a meaningful connection spans from abusive parents to high school mean girls, from dominating bosses to manipulative spouses, and everything in between. Regardless of the intensity and magnitude of each conflictual dynamic, the continuum of possibilities in which relationships can cause problems in our lives is both broad and deep.

You have likely experienced the double bind of meaning and challenge that comes in the package of relationships—especially those that are more intimate. Maybe you are currently walking the tightrope between indecision and decision about whether to leave an unhealthy relationship that you have been unsure about for a while. By now, you probably realize the profound ways we influence and are influenced by each other. And you may have found it's not always for the better. When you share a dynamic with another human being—be they your partner, friend, mother-in-law, or bank teller—you no longer exist alone in your own universe. The inclusion of another person's array of needs, desires, projections, and behaviors factors into the delicate interplay that influences your interactions and associations. This is the dance of relationships. A particular sensitivity and attunement are required to adapt, flow, and respond to the natural give and take between two people who care for one another.

But what happens when the care for each other gets distorted and causes more damage than nourishment? Maybe you don't feel quite so cared for anymore, or you are coming to realize that you never did in one or many of the relationships you have endured. Maybe it feels like time for a relationship revolution within your own life where you reclaim your worth and value and selectively give your heart only to those who treat you with kindness that requires no justification.

As you will learn, there are times to dig in, times to get out, times to back off, and times to lean in. There is no standardized approach to the intricacies of every relationship, but there are patterns that become evident when you hone your attention. At the core of each teaching and story within this book you will find three threads weaving throughout healthy dynamics (and missing from unhealthy ones): honesty, kindness, and respect. These are the *three gates* of healthy relationships. They determine whether you feel grace or chaos in your connections. This is true regardless of whether you foster a repair with someone or say goodbye to them. You will learn the nuance necessary for thoughtful relationship cultivation, maintenance, and termination and understand how sometimes your unresolved personal issues are the culprit in a harmful dynamic.

Throughout the text I will write about the choice point between whether to *mend* or *move on*—hang on to a relationship with the grit to salvage it or get honest about its hopelessness and break free. You will also come to fully understand what is involved in each trajectory. You may have chosen this book because you know something doesn't feel quite right in your relationship (or many of your relationships), but you still need to discern exactly how injurious—or even toxic—it truly is. The book will help by first familiarizing you with the *seven traps of toxic relationships*, which illuminate the mindsets that may be keeping you stuck in dysfunctional dynamics. The traps are these:

1. **Buy-in:** Accepting beliefs, values, and behaviors of a toxic person or family without questioning whether they are aligned with and healthy for you.
2. **Comfort:** Prioritizing the comfort of others over your own mental health and well-being.

3. **Powerlessness:** Surrendering power by allowing yourself to be manipulated, gaslit, and abused.

4. **False ownership:** Considering yourself to be "the problem" and allowing all blame for the relationship's issues to fall on you as the scapegoat.

5. **Unhealed trauma:** Allowing inner wounds to fuel the repetition of destructive patterns in one or many relationships.

6. **Avoidance:** Making excuses, living in denial, and hoping that relationships will improve with time without facing the root problem.

7. **Codependency:** Forming codependent bonds with others and believing it is the same as genuine connection and love.

It is important to explore the hidden ways toxicity can lurk inside long-standing relationships when your drive for human connection attracts and sustains bonds that have been built on unhealthy foundations. The *seven traps* will help you identify when the bittersweetness of troubled relationships is far more *bitter* than *sweet*. Then your soul-searching will begin as you come to recognize damaging patterns such as resentment, betrayal, self-abandonment, and others that have negatively contributed to the relational pain and suffering you experience. At this point, you will learn how to navigate the *mend* or *move on* fork in the road and come to clearly understand what each path involves. By using the same techniques I have taught for decades to hundreds of therapy clients, you will get crystal clear about how toxic is too toxic.

If you come to find that the relationship(s) where you have the most difficulty are worth *mending*, the coming pages will provide you with a path to authentic repair that will up-level your communication and behavioral tools through greater self-awareness, accountability, and deeper connection to foster healing. The exploration of depth psychology will prompt inner reflection, help you cease unhealthy patterns, and redirect your bonds toward restoration you can feel great about. This approach will guide you toward self-realization and integrity-testing that leads you to seek wisdom from the state of your nervous system and notice parts of yourself that may have been pretzeling to fit in misaligned relationships that were locked into destructive habits.

If you discern that the healthiest trajectory for your mind, heart, body, and soul is to *move on* from a harmful dynamic (or multiple dynamics) that show no hope for improvement, you're in good hands. This triumphant approach will help you walk away with self-respect from relationships that have infused your life with harm and cruelty. The chapters ahead will help you navigate the messy limbo you may have felt entrapped within for years or even decades and find a way out. By coming to accept when a connection is beyond repair (when trust and emotional or physical safety have been tampered with to the point of no return), you will learn how to disentangle from destructive people once and for all. You will find an expansive toolkit to help you cut ties with anyone who harms you—even if they are a close family member or longtime friend—by incorporating boundary work, art therapy to bring the unconscious into awareness, and practices to build clarity and fortitude. Stepping out of dark dynamics toward the light of a hopeful future without toxic bonds is within reach.

I want you to know that I am with you on this complex and heart-wrenching topic. I too am a survivor of intergenerational trauma and systemic abuse and dysfunction from a profoundly toxic family. It is my hope that the personal stories I share in the pages to come will feel relatable and allow you to see yourself in these experiences. Anecdotes from my own experiences with toxic family members and friends combined with case studies from my clients who have navigated potent relational ruptures, repairs, and endings will help you learn how to prioritize your psychological health and safety. You will come to see how your tendency toward politeness and people-pleasing may have preserved safety in your relationships, but it also may have kept vicious patterns alive in your family and social groups for generations.

If you are seeking a book that will help you contort and conform within the confines of a toxic relationship, you're in the wrong place. This book isn't about making a destructive relationship work. It's about recognizing when a poisonous connection will not improve and learning how to break free from it with dignity—even if that means cutting off someone you have felt close to for most (or all) of your life. Together, let's identify the noxious qualities of toxic relationships and advocate for ourselves and each other—understanding that nobody deserves to be treated in ways that continuously dehumanize, confuse, or wound them. When it comes to relationships, if they can't be deeply healed, perhaps they should be left behind.

You may have noticed in recent years that there has been a rising willingness within society to cut ties with toxic relationships. I strongly believe that this is more than just a trend, as your estranged mother may claim from her soapbox. I see it as a powerful step forward for individuals and the collective. Here are some statistics that reflect where so many people stand these days with their toxic family members, friends, and colleagues:

They're fed up and actively seeking help to either salvage what can be healed or close the door on those too entrenched in their dysfunction to change.

For starters, "toxic" was the Oxford English Dictionary's word of the year in 2018,[1] and "gaslighting" was Merriam-Webster's choice in 2022.[2] Additionally, #ToxicFamily has surpassed 1.9 billion TikTok views.[3] Shocking new data indicates a remarkable shift in how modern people relate to their closest connections. One study[4] shows that almost 30 percent of Americans over the age of eighteen have broken up with a family member, and 11 percent of mothers are estranged from an adult child who cut ties with them.[5] Another study revealed that 80 percent of participants who closed the door on dysfunctional family members reported positive outcomes from this choice.[6]

In nonfamilial relationships,[7] three-quarters of US employees report having a "toxic" boss, and 84 percent of women and 75 percent of men have had a toxic friend. Nearly 85 percent of survey takers maintained a poisonous friendship beyond the bounds of "healthy" because friend breakups are so hard.[8] Meanwhile, influential sources like Oprah, *The Atlantic,* and the *Today* show have recently aired stories on the prevalence of family and friendship breakups.

The data is clear, and to me that reflects the clarity of our society that we need to push back against generations-old clichés that are considered truisms like "blood is thicker than water" and "family is family, no matter what." They're simply untrue in some cases, and the time has come to face that reality with a willingness to change.

To my knowledge, *Mend or Move On* is the first book on toxic relationships to be written by a licensed psychotherapist who is also a board-certified art therapist. I have a feeling you are going to love my innovative approach to self-understanding and healing that integrates creativity, science, and psychology. You will learn how to tap into the exquisite intelligence that lies in wait beneath the surface of your consciousness with creativity as a guiding light. Your nervous system will feel more regulated, and you will source from the wisdom of your physiology to develop a road map that leads you toward a bright future of relationships that support and nourish you. Through an Internal Family Systems (IFS) "parts psychology" lens,[9] you will come to know the parts of yourself that have been striving to protect you while other more fragile parts have been exiled in their woundedness. To support your integration of the topics we will cover, each chapter provides How-To Tips, which are artistic prompts and inquisitive questions I brainstormed to inspire profound self-examination and insight. These offerings will help you apply this meaningful work to your own life by implementing practical tools and considerations in your journal, sketchbook, conversations with loved ones, and musings in your own headspace.

Here, you will be supported in the life-reclaiming journey of finally exiting the seductive loop of venomous relationships that take far more than they give. You will be empowered to salvage bonds that show hope for repair and walk away from anyone who continuously harms you. By the final page, you will be equipped to confidently break free from *toxic* and attract future relationships that are healthy, joyful, and soul nourishing. Are you ready to delve in? Let's go.

CHAPTER 1

Relationships Are Like Oil Paintings

Oil painting has never been my thing. Maybe the part of me that prefers certainty is squeamish with the ongoing flexibility inherent in the medium. You see, depending on how thickly oil paint is applied, it can take a very (very, very) long time to dry. In fact, Van Gogh's *The Starry Night*, painted in 1889, is rumored to have wet paint in certain areas to this day, though I cannot confirm if this is true. Suffice it to say that oil paint takes a while to dry, especially if it is layered thickly. Relationships share this quality, but I would venture to say that they are even more extreme: If relationships were oil paintings, they would *never* dry.

Relationships are constant works in progress; they are never complete. They do not arrive at a final state of being where they remain forevermore, like the stillness achieved by acrylic paint or a drawing made with pen and ink. For days, years, and decades, relationships remain malleable. They can be smudged and enhanced, and layers can be concealed and scraped away. At any phase, a murky mess can be made from what was previously beautiful. For this reason, we should be unsurprised when relational dynamics shift, change, and morph into new iterations of themselves. In many cases, the layering and thoughtful reworking results in finely tuned bonds and—dare I say—masterpieces. Conversely, other dynamics are more like an overworked oil painting; all that's left to do with the mess is discard it once and for all and start fresh.

As the cocreator of a perplexing relationship, you must discern and clarify if the continuous work in progress of your affiliation with another is worth maintaining. You may find that your connection holds the potential to transform into a marvel, or you may discover that its inner workings are destroyed to the extent that necessitates it being tossed. According to the basic principles of art therapy, different creative materials hold the power to align metaphorically with a person's emotional experiences. Just as oil paint can mirror the wet, layered quality of one relationship, so can colored pencil represent the control and precision that may be imperative in another dynamic. The flesh-like quality of clay can create an opportunity for an artist to work through physical trauma that involved the body, and the drippy nature of watercolor can allow a person to gain more comfort with messiness, mistakes, and feeling out of control. When the metaphorical dimensions of art therapy are used to support your relational healing process, you find more emotional ground to explore and different ways to navigate embedded experiences and patterns. The expressive process of creativity also has neurological effects on the brain that wire and rewire our behaviors, default thinking, and engagement with our lives based on the experiences we live through[1]—including our relational dynamics.

You read in the introduction about the *mend* or *move on* choice point, where you must discern whether a relationship is worthwhile enough to justify hunkering down and pouring reparative energy into or if it has tipped so far into harmful territory that it is unlikely ever to change and thus must end. In oil paintings, as in relationships, you may reach a point where you must decide if you want to dig your heels in and *mend* the painting or if you should cut your losses, preserve your sanity, and start anew.

The *mend* or *move on* choice point can happen when a relationship simply grows misaligned, and it can also happen when toxicity is present. Perhaps you have grown to realize that your connection has always had undercurrents of dysfunction and poisonous qualities that you only recently have refused to tolerate. Maybe your relationship has grown toxic over time. Regardless of its path and process, toxic is toxic, and I would never recommend that a person grit their teeth and settle for an unhealthy bond that undermines their autonomy, shunts their strength, or belittles their value—particularly when the relationship shows no hope for improvement.

If you know *toxic*, you may recognize some of these statements that people trapped in dynamics like these tend to whisper to themselves within their own psyches for years or decades. These are some of the stories you might tell yourself that keep you ensnared:

- They will change in time. I just need to wait it out.
- It's not that bad. I am just too sensitive.
- I know there's a good heart in there. They don't mean it.
- My expectations are unrealistic. No relationship is perfect.
- This is just how our family is. (Or the workplace. Or the social world.)
- Everyone has issues. You don't walk away from family.
- I just have to grow a thicker skin.

> **How-To Tip** Write down all of your narratives in your journal. Include any from my list that resonate with you, and add others that are unique to your experience. Take a long, brave look at the stories you have been telling yourself about your unhealthy relationship(s), and then write about how sitting with those dysfunctional justifications makes you feel.

If any of the narratives from my list sound familiar, or if you can identify others I didn't mention, you have been gaslighting yourself. You likely did this because it was adaptive—meaning it helped you stay safe, earn belonging, or secure love in some way that felt imperative to your survival. Even so, you have been manipulating your perception of reality and the truth in order to stay comfortable, safe, or compliant in a dynamic that may be or has been unhealthy for you for far too long. You have been working and reworking an oil painting that likely cannot be salvaged, just making a plain ol' mess rather than a work of wonder. Especially if you have been self-reflective in truthful ways, explored your unhealed wounds and patterns in therapy, had many difficult conversations that did not result in healthy shifts in the relationship, and stuck around for years or decades hoping for improvement without seeing it manifest, it's time to leave.

One sneaky trait of many poisonous relationships is that they can muddle your mind, your heart, and even your body's internal compass of morality. Envision a painting where the colors and subjects have become so inextricably overworked that all you can see is a smear of ugly browns. Paintings like these often have too many layers and have been churned around by the artist's hand to the point of no return. Similarly, rather than aiming for a clear and bright picture, toxic relationships hide their destructive undercurrents beneath layers of fear, misunderstanding, and emotional warfare like shame and blame. This especially happens within families or systems that weaponize secrecy, prize power, and wield manipulation and control as though they were magic wands. They insidiously plant confusion about whether you should *mend* or *move on*. More than anything else, this conflictual feeling of indecision is what often ultimately leads people to gain the clarity they need to cut out toxic parents, siblings, friends, and partners. Maybe it's what led you to this book.

Awakening to the unacceptability of warped relational lenses is more than a trend. It is not impulsive, irrational, or unfounded, as those you choose to break up with may claim. In fact, most often when a person seeks a resource like this book to support their healthy movement away from toxic people, they have tried everything and anything possible to avoid reaching this end. They have endured more than anyone deserves, attempted repair innumerable times, and reached a devastating understanding that often feels like a health ultimatum: me or them.

When the metaphorical messy oil painting (ahem, relationship) cannot continue for a moment longer, the painting must be discarded. This can be tricky business because society and many of its outdated traditional narratives about family and friendship would have you believe that the right thing to do is to either learn to like the muddy brown your relationship has become or continue to tirelessly mix, layer, and obscure the truth of your relational painting without ever considering the option that you can just stop.

> **How-To Tip**   Grab some paints and paper or canvas, and give this a try. Blend, layer, and overwork your image until your blues, yellows, reds, and all other colors become an unsightly mess of brown. Notice how it feels to overdo and overmix to this extent, and become aware of the emotions that arise within you. Do you feel disgusted? Hopeless? Angry with yourself? Frustrated with the paint? For further processing, write about your experience in your journal.

The thing about brown muddy messes of mixed paint is that what's done cannot be undone. You cannot extricate blue and orange from brown and backtrack to more pleasing dynamics between the colors. When you realize you cannot bring the vivid hues back from the mess of your relationship and you dislike the brown you mixed, you then must consider the *how* and *why* of letting it go.

Though the mess of relationships cannot be rewound, some dynamics can build a new reality from the remains of the old. One way this can look, in paint terms, would be to plant sequins in the mess of brown and bedazzle a new dynamic with intention and care. This is not always possible, as you well know if you have attempted relational bedazzlement for years and somehow the mess remains.

If you reach a place where you are just done and you have nothing left to give a relationship that seems doomed, it's natural to experience fear, shame, or inner conflict about going against the grain and walking away from someone you once loved. Making and accepting your decision takes time and intention, and it certainly requires the bravery to counter your prior ways of thinking and rework your core beliefs. If you stay the course, you will likely come to understand that courageously closing the door on a bond that wounds you is not a weakness or meanness. In fact, it indicates that you are in the midst of a powerful growth spurt that will benefit you individually while also positively changing the trajectory of your own lineage by disrupting patterns of intergenerational trauma. When you heal your ancestral line by making healthy relational choices and saying no to abuse and dysfunction, you contribute to healing the entire collective of society.

You make ripples with every behavior and shift you integrate within yourself. By saying *this ends here* or *stop this now*, your empowerment extends further than you could imagine. Your children and their children will feel the uplifting effects of your choice to stop tolerating maltreatment. Even strangers you may never meet might catch wind of your growth and feel its benefits through the ripples you set into motion with your actions, behaviors, and words. Just imagine, if your children witness you courageously disrupting dysfunctional patterns, they will be more likely to uphold healthy expectations and behaviors in their relationships. From there, others they connect with will experience health, balance, and respect as they benefit from a chain reaction you set into motion that continues for generations forward. You have the power to model positive interpersonal dynamics for others and affect change far beyond yourself with the choices you make and the actions you take.

The term *butterfly effect*[2] was coined by Edward Lorenz at the 139th meeting of the American Association for the Advancement of Science when he posed the following question: "Does the flap of a butterfly's wings in Brazil set off a tornado in Texas?" Of course a butterfly does not have the power to directly stir up a tornado, but it can set in motion a string of events that may ultimately grow infinitely larger than itself as it participates in the interconnected web of all things. By representing the power of a tiny change in the homeostasis of a larger system, the butterfly effect explains how one delicate action can impact monumental change beyond itself in ways it may never come to understand or realize.

CHAPTER 2

The Skull and Crossbones of Toxic Relationships

When I think of the word "toxic," I visualize a skull and crossbones and noxious green smoke rising from a contraband science beaker. The very word surfaces the following associations in my consciousness: corrosive, poisonous, caustic, destructive, and deadly. Although this kind of venomous experience can be sparked between conflicting elements of the periodic table, it has also become a term to describe relationships that fester, bubble, and ooze like poison.

The term "toxic relationships" has received massive attention in recent years. The buzz reached the extent that the term "gaslighting" was named word of the year in 2022 by Merriam-Webster, America's oldest dictionary publisher.[1] We will circle back to gaslighting later, but if the term is new to you here's a brief definition: Gaslighting is a harmful and dangerous form of emotional manipulation that makes a person question their reality. Phrases like "you don't really feel that way" or "you're too sensitive" fall in the ballpark of gaslighting. A word earns the acclaim of being the "word of the year" when it is searched most frequently, out of all English words, throughout a given year. In 2022, Merriam-Webster's award reflected society's awareness of toxicity in relationships as demonstrated by the collective relatability to the word "gaslighting."

> **How-To Tip**   Muse on how you feel about pop psychology
> buzzwords you may have seen (ad nauseum) online, in your
> social media feeds, in the media, or even at a casual happy
> hour with your colleagues. What do words like these bring up
> for you? If you feel inclined to be creative, use magazine
> clippings or online images of psychology buzzwords to create
> a collage that represents how you feel about these words.
> Perhaps part of your collage represents areas in life where the
> buzzwords are positive and helpful while another part of your
> collage represents how the words can be detrimental.

When something becomes a buzzword, it is important not
to use it informally but instead to remain conscious of its true
definition and implications despite its popularity. As awareness
of "toxic relationships" and "gaslighting" continues to spread
like wildfire throughout society, it is important to understand
something: A relationship that feels frustrating, icky, uncomfortable, or unsatisfactory is not necessarily toxic. There are
shades of misalignment that can occur in relationships that may
or may not be genuinely toxic. Although it can feel satisfying to
label something (or someone) "toxic" when you feel annoyed or
irked, I encourage you to remember this: All toxic relationships
are misaligned, but not all misaligned relationships are toxic.
The truth is, it's easy to call another person "toxic" when you
are not getting what you need. This is where blame and victimization come in, and they are two land mines that can irrevoca-
bly weaken the integrity of a relationship. Let's go there. . . .

Blame and Victimization

I'll start this section by loudly and clearly stating for all to hear
that YES, there are circumstances of victimization that are horrific and unspeakable. More often than anyone wants to admit,
situations exist where people experience awful abuse and mal-

treatment that most certainly places them in a lower position of power and in certain danger with an unsafe person. Physical, mental, sexual, verbal, and psychological abuse are undeniably present around our globe, and they have profoundly negative consequences on the bodies, minds, and spirits of those who fall victim to such maltreatment. Victimization is very real, and there are countless people in dire situations who need help and rescuing from unthinkable abuse.

Like most topics in the complex, messy territory of relationships, there exists a continuum of severity when it comes to blame and victimization. Words such as these can easily become misused, misconstrued, and distorted, so we must all use caution with how we wield them. The range of severity of victimization spans from unthinkable abuse on one end to using the term "victim" in ways that are psychologically warped and meant to shunt personal accountability on the extreme other end, and every shade between. We will further discuss the various manifestations of abuse in the pages to come, but this section hones in on how a person can consciously or unconsciously weaponize victimization to project blame, avoid responsibility, or manipulate the perception of a situation.

True victimization is quite different from the convenient adaptation of the word to punish, scapegoat, or condemn another out of hurt feelings or wounded pride. Mainly this tends to highlight a person's emotional attachment to needing to feel *right* in a particular circumstance by making the other person *wrong*. People play this game for a myriad of reasons, often to counterbalance their lack of accountability for the sinking ship their relationship has become.

Identifying as a victim is not *wrong* or *right*. It is a position of weakness, opposite to someone stronger and more powerful, that renders a person helpless in their own life. Rarely is someone truly powerless once they become a developed adult, but in order to grow beyond victim identification they must willingly find the inner strength, courage, and conviction to take aligned action for change.

Terry Real coined the term "offending from the victim."[2] This is when someone who has identified themselves as a victim (even if only in their own mind) feels justified in harming another person to balance the scales. It's when a person feels weak and helpless and from that position behaves violently or aggressively like an offender. Such behavior often pairs with a narrative like *you wounded me, so it's okay for me to wound you deeper.* Such an inclination is a psychologically distorted form of revenge built upon emotional violence rather than compassionate repair. It is not true victimhood and can cause immeasurable damage in both a relationship and a person's psyche.

In truth, getting even is rarely as satisfying as people imagine it will be. It mostly leaves a person feeling guilty and ashamed of their own abusive behavior rather than feeling as though the scales of justice have been leveled. I often tell my young kids that being mean to someone who was mean to you first only makes two mean people—and that's not who you are. Counter-abuse is quite the same. It turns out that the best revenge possible is to peacefully move on with your life and leave your abuser in the dust. The *take the high road* and *be the bigger person* teachings from childhood do actually hold a golden nugget of wisdom when it comes to walking away from perpetrators without inadvertently becoming one yourself.

> **How-To Tip**   Journal about your internal reaction to the words "victim" and "perpetrator." Notice what associations, feeling, judgments, or reactions arise in you. For an added art therapeutic element, create character sketches of "The Victim" and "The Perpetrator" by exploring the shapes, colors,

and lines that resonate with each of their energetics. Notice if your character sketches are aligned with how society views these archetypes or if you experience them differently from your mass culture.

The following examples describe two different relationships that abruptly and painfully ended due to differing needs between my client Sonya and two others in her life. These are examples of nonabusive relationships that grew to become warped projections one might call "toxic," but in fact they were really just misaligned. At the time, both breakups were deeply uncomfortable for my client. The multiple conversations during our sessions about problematic dynamics in both scenarios were heavy topics involving much angst and avoidance. Thanks to these ruptures, Sonya has now experienced being on both sides of the relational coin, so to speak. In one circumstance Sonya behaved as the coldly resistant participant while in the other she was needy and smothering. In our sessions, Sonya has explained that she now has a fuller experience of growth from living through both scenarios.

Here's what happened: The first relationship (a friendship) had been afloat for about two years. For most of the time Sonya felt a tense resistance that she had never been fully honest about with herself or the other person (let's call her Judy). Something felt misaligned from the relationship's inception, but at the time Sonya lacked the skills and ego strength to say "thanks but no thanks" to the other person's pursuit of connection. Over time, Judy increased her expectations for the role she envisioned Sonya should play in her life, the intimacy she demanded, and the time and energy she needed from Sonya to fulfill her needs. Sonya mostly complied, which was a mistake she made by self-abandoning and ignoring her gut instinct that the relationship was askew. Lacking integrity and honesty, Sonya led Judy to believe that she was on board with Judy's assumptions about the quality and intensity of their connection. Eventually, as always, the truth came out. Sonya's discomfort with coercing herself to give more than she wanted to give bubbled to the surface in a series of two or three conversations where she expressed her unwillingness to show up the way Judy demanded.

It took the repetition of these conversations for Sonya to fully express her need for *less* while Judy expressed her need for *more*. The misfit dynamic Sonya and Judy had cocreated and sustained was evident to Sonya, but Judy never seemed to reach that understanding. All she could perceive was Sonya's rejection and her pain as though it were as simple as A + B = C. Needless to say, their ending was turbulent but ultimately necessary. At the time, Sonya thought Judy was *toxic*. The way Judy related to Sonya certainly felt uncomfortable. Sonya felt cornered, coerced, and required to invest effort, energy, love, and time she did not freely offer. Sonya had defined her discomfort as a response to *toxicity* at that time, but now she sees that it was simply a relational incongruity between divergent people with wildly oppositional needs and boundaries. There was no danger, no abuse, and nothing Sonya couldn't walk away, heal, and completely recover from.

Years later, Sonya found herself on the flip side of her prior experience in a conversation with a different friend about a relationship that had endured for longer than ten years. Through the natural ebb and flow of connection, their relationship had moved in and out of emotional intimacy during various periods of their lives. Discontent arrived, however, when the friendship's closeness steeply dropped off in a way that left Sonya feeling acutely disconnected. Where there was once warmth, things felt cold. Sonya was the one who reached out for connection most of the time, if not exclusively. When she shared her need for deeper connection, Sonya was met with resistance similar to what she herself had emanated years earlier toward Judy. Now it seemed Sonya was the needy one opposite a person who couldn't or wouldn't meet her emotional needs. As she processed this rupture in our sessions, Sonya wondered if this person considered her to be *toxic*, as she had thought Judy was.

The juxtaposition between these two dwindling relationships was striking then, and still is, as a series of opportunities for my client to experience being both the smotherer and the one who feels smothered. We will never know the perspective of either friend from these relationships and whether they would identify their dynamics with Sonya as *toxic*, but Sonya came to realize in our work that neither relationship actually was. Despite hurtful energetics that ensued for all involved, the relationships simply reached misalignment too immense for continuation.

> **How-To Tip**   Consider a relationship of yours that went south. Did you consider it toxic? Maybe you were labeled toxic at the time, or you thought of the other person as such. How do you feel about it now after time has passed? Explore this in your journal.

Now that we have discussed painful (yet nontoxic) relational undercurrents, let's define what makes a genuinely toxic relationship *toxic*.[3] My definition is threefold. In order for a relationship to be truly toxic, not just misaligned, it must be all of the following:

- *Consistent and persistent:* Toxic relationships are more than just one-off experiences. There can certainly be toxic behaviors that spring up sporadically here or there, but without the harmful words, actions, or conduct occurring regularly, the relationship does not qualify as toxic. "Consistency and persistence" means that the destructive energetics continue over time in repetition so that they become cycles or patterns, not just singular events.

- *Truly harmful or showing the potential to become so:* Toxic relationships harm your mind, body, heart, or entire being in very real ways. Sometimes the harm caused by a venomous person is visible, like the bruises an abuser leaves after they physically injure someone. In other cases, toxicity can be more challenging to identify because it appears invisible but can be strongly felt emotionally or energetically, as in cases of emotional abuse, manipulation and gaslighting, brainwashing and psychological warfare, and other such dangerous behaviors. Toxic relationships are abusive and caustic. If your self-esteem is dismantled, your body or mind feels violated, your free will is caged, or your emotions feel snowplowed, it's toxic. In scenarios where a relationship shows the potential to become toxic, you may not presently experience the violence of a person's toxicity, but you might sense it coming. This happens when you witness their use of poisonous behaviors toward someone else, when they tell stories of past relationships where they behaved in toxic ways, or when they show signs of upping the ante and escalating their behaviors in the direction of true toxicity. Your spidey sense, gut feeling, intuition, or whatever else you may call your inner compass will tell you when a person's behavior doesn't match their true Self. If they appear kind and charming but your stomach is churning and your mind feels skeptical, keep a close eye on what those messages might be telling you.

- *Twisty-turny, pushy-pully:* Okay, so it's not a technical scientific term, but it's a good description of how a toxic relationship feels in the body, somatically. Toxic relationships are confusing. They mess with you. It feels like a game, but one you don't know the rules for. One moment you're happy, but soon after you're sobbing. You feel secure, then you're unsure if the floor might drop out from beneath you. One day you are their favorite person, but two weeks later they are avoiding you. Keeping up with the mind warp of a toxic relationship is exhausting and perplexing, to say the least. If you feel in your mind, heart, and body that twisty-turny, pushy-pully sensation, the relationship is probably toxic.

Toxicity can exist in partnerships, marriages, friendships, work relationships, and family relationships. As a survivor of a toxic family system, Dr. Sherrie Campbell teaches in-depth about the numerous complexities of living with toxic family members. She also teaches how to free yourself from malignant familial relationships in her several wonderful books.[4] A relationship that operates from a toxic foundation has cruelty, malice, or harmful energetics at its core. Often such interplay is unconscious and related to a person's unhealed trauma and personal wounding. The saying "hurt people hurt people" applies in situations like this. A person may not directly intend to harm their partner, friend, employee, or loved one, but they cannot see past the veil of their own pain and suffering to understand that they are infusing the connection with profound dysfunction. In other more dangerous scenarios with psychologically unwell people, toxic treatment can be conscious and intentional. These are displays of malicious toxicity from those with covert agendas for power, control, or dominance and individuals who prey on others for personal gain. On a deep level, "hurt people hurt people" also applies here because those who intentionally harm others almost certainly operate from a worldview built from experiences that taught them some form of brutality firsthand.

Gaslighting

Whether conscious or unconscious, intentional or not, forms of psychological manipulation, dangerous behavior, and abuse of any kind qualify a relationship as toxic. Once a relationship accrues the criteria where it can be considered *toxic*, it would best serve all involved for it to swiftly and completely end. One particularly toxic trait of many unhealthy relationships, especially those with individuals who display narcissistic traits or narcissistic personality disorder, is gaslighting. It wasn't named the word of the year for nothing—the use of this manipulative control strategy is more pervasive than anyone wants to believe. "Gaslighting" is when someone plants seeds of doubt or uncertainty in your psyche with shame, guilt, blame, or accusations that cause you to question what you know to be true. Here are examples of gaslighting statements:

- You don't really feel that way.
- You're too sensitive.
- I never did that.
- You have no idea what you're talking about.
- You remember it wrong.
- This is all because of you.

- You're crazy! You're sick in the head if you think that.
- You know I would never hurt you. I did that because I love you.
- It's not that bad. Other people have it so much worse.

Gaslighting can be used both consciously and unconsciously to shift blame onto another person in the service of avoiding responsibility or accountability. In psychology this behavior is called "deflection." It is an avoidance strategy that keeps one person in the *right* by firmly placing another in the *wrong*. To fuel the master plan, a gaslighter aims to convince the other person to see themselves as wrong to cause confusion and spark an emotional collapse that ultimately fulfills the gaslighter's needs. Make no mistake, gaslighting is a form of psychological and emotional abuse. Repeated exposure to someone who uses gaslighting as a tool for control, power, and defense undoubtedly wounds deeply. This can open the gateway for additional relational toxicity such as enmeshment, codependency, insecurity, resentment, and deep-seated fear and unease.

A common emotionally manipulative behavior (and form of gaslighting) is what psychologists term "love bombing." This happens when a perpetrator heaps on heavy doses of attention, complements, and gushing adoration in a calculated manner designed to disarm your defenses by making you feel desirable. You may become confused by love bombing because it is not a consistent state of connection and belonging between yourself and another but rather a strategic tool used to mess with your beliefs about how lovable you are. Love bombing is a manipulative waterfall of over-the-top gestures, efforts, behaviors, and actions that overwhelm a person with attention and sticky-sweet love-like messages. It doesn't last for long because the amount of energy it takes to pummel someone with love is exhausting, so

as soon as the love bomber gains what they set out to achieve—
be it your compliance, a favor you didn't originally want to
give, or anything else they sought from you—the love disappears, and you are left cold and empty in its wake, wondering
what just happened and why you feel so used. Love bombing is
used by psychopathic, sociopathic, and narcissistic people, and
those with other personality disorders (as well as others in dysfunctional relationships) as a tool to control and distort the way
they are perceived and ultimately get what they want. Love
bombing is not legitimate love. It is a saccharine-sweet, honey-
laced agenda for manipulation and dominance to get something from someone, sway a person into their favor, or secure a
relationship that might be drifting beyond their control.

It is never okay for another person to toy with your mind
and heart or tell you how you feel in any given situation. You are
entitled to your unique experiences. If someone expresses curiosity about your position, you may choose to share your
opinion; however, they do not have the right to coerce you into
believing something you feel is untrue. When there is a power
differential between people, such as a parent/child dynamic or
a spousal partnership where one person holds more control
and command, the asymmetry provides a distinct contrast
that places one person in greater vulnerability than the other.
This is fertile ground for gaslighting to take root if someone
with authority takes advantage of their position. It can take
years to unpack the damage this type of manipulation creates
because it attacks a person's identity and self-trust at a deep
level. Repeated exposure to treatment like this can impact a
person to the point where they don't know who they are, what
they believe, or what or whom they can trust.

In addition to seeing manipulative behavior like gaslighting
in your personal relationships, you will also notice it in books,

movies, and the media. Something I admire about novelist Jodi Picoult is the factual information she includes in her books on a variety of topics. One thing I learned from Picoult's 2022 novel *Mad Honey*[5] is that a certain type of honey exists that should never be eaten. Different from the nourishing honey known to be healthy and beneficial for our bodies, there is a much more dangerous varietal called "mad honey" that has quite the opposite effect. Mad honey is created by bees that collect nectar from particular flora filled with poisonous grayanotoxins.[6] This sweet poison has been used in biological warfare since 399 BC because it causes a battery of harmful symptoms in the human body that can even be fatal if left untreated. The feeding and ingestion of mad honey is eerily similar, in the context of relationships, to a manipulator working their magic on an unsuspecting person who trusts them. As Picoult writes, "The secret weapon of mad honey, of course, is that you expect it to be sweet, not deadly. . . . By the time it messes with your head, with your heart, it's too late."[7] If you speak to a person who has been profoundly or repeatedly abused with gaslighting or manipulation, they likely understand how a person can seem sweet only to later be discovered to be inherently toxic—and even dangerous.

Emotional manipulation is like an optical illusion but for the heart and psyche rather than the eyes. Optical illusions are fascinating. Maybe you recall seeing an image of a vase that morphs into to conversing faces when you soften your gaze and blink. There was a famed dress that spread virally online when viewers realized that not everyone saw the same colors when looking at the image (some people saw a gold and white dress while others saw a blue and black one). Another example of an optical illusion is the beautiful image of a young woman's profile that suddenly shape-shifts to become an old lady's face when the viewer looks again. Optical illusions are incredibly similar to the distorted perception of a person who has been emotionally manipulated. This person has the uncanny experience of thinking they know the reality of a situation only to feel flickering doubt when they look again, realize that their perception was warped, and become aware of the existence of another possibility they never previously imagined. The vacillation back and forth can be quite confusing, leading a person to feel unsure about reality and even uncertain about their sanity. A skillful manipulator knows how to prey on someone experiencing such confusion by weaving a convincing web of illusion that projects a mirage suited to the needs and desires of the manipulator. Such tactics are immensely believable despite how colossally the deception differs from objective truth.

> **How-To Tip**   Write about a time when you were manipulated by someone. Did it feel like mad honey or an optical illusion? Explain. Next, consider a time when you were manipulative. From the perspective of the manipulator, can you now see that you may have been serving mad honey to someone? Write about this experience from your present vantage point.

If you have been in a toxic relationship (or many of them), you understand the unnatural push-pull feeling of being both connected to and repelled by a person you had hoped to sustain a meaningful relationship with. Unfortunately, relational dynamics with malignant intentions have existed in humanity for longer than modern researchers can fully study, and these dynamics will likely persist into the future. It simply seems to be part of the mortal experience that humans have the capacity for such dynamics, and it seems equally pertinent that we learn to healthfully navigate them. Only you can moderate your exposure to such harmful dynamics. Each time you move away from a person or connection that feels toxic, you reinforce your self-trust that you can make sound relational choices that protect and honor you. Let this chapter be a reminder of the power you hold within to steer toward relationships that foster health and well-being in your heart, soul, body, and mind.

CHAPTER 3

The Seven Traps of Toxic Relationships

Sometimes a person enters a new relationship, be it with a friend, a colleague, or anyone else, and they have that spidey sense from the get-go that something is not right. In other instances, a person is born into a family with one or many toxic relationships, and they grow to realize just how unhealthy the connections truly are. In yet other scenarios, a person suddenly awakens to the recognition that a dynamic they have cocreated with another is laced with dysfunctional patterns and behaviors that simply must stop. Regardless of how people come to realize that a relationship they're in is toxic, many experience feeling trapped in a sticky snare that seems complicated to extricate from. This often happens because toxic relationships tend to weaponize emotions like blame and fear, which can perpetuate codependent and avoidant behaviors that feel cyclical in nature. When you're caught in a loop like this, you might feel so consumed by the drama (and subsequent self-protection) that is necessary to survive the dynamic that you lack the ability to find a way out of it.

In my clinical work with therapy clients across different social, behavioral, and age groups, I have identified *seven traps* that are consistently reported as being the most dominant culprits that block people from relational health and freedom. This chapter will plant seeds for your reflective inquiry. As the book unfolds and takes you deeper into these insights, these seeds will grow into blooms of awareness that support healthy transformation for your relationships. Each of the *seven traps* is larger than this chapter can contain. Rather than a point-and-shoot breakdown of all problems and solutions related to toxic relationships, these traps will lay the framework for following chapters that discuss in far more detail the snares that contribute to your entrapment. For now, think of this chapter as a sampler platter that identifies some of the major problems toxic relationships usher into our lives, including a brief breakdown of the three facets that contribute to how each trap ensnares people. For each trap you will learn three things:

- How to identify and recognize the jaws of a trap in action
- How to disentangle from the grip of a trap that has you in its claws
- How to avoid repeatedly getting hooked by the trap in the future

Here they are, folks, the traps that tie people up in knots in relationships that harm them and destroy their sense of identity, sovereignty, autonomy, and well-being:

1. Buy-in
2. Comfort
3. Powerlessness
4. False ownership
5. Unhealed trauma
6. Avoidance
7. Codependency

Ready? Let's go. Take a deep breath, and let's tackle these traps one at a time.

Trap #1: Buy-In

The jaws of "buy-in" in action: Accepting the beliefs, values, and behaviors of a toxic person or family without questioning whether they are aligned and healthy for you.

Your participation is central to whether or not a toxic person can play out a dysfunctional dynamic with you. Your attention and compliance fuel your conscious or unconscious willingness to participate in a relationship on their terms. Toxic individuals love nothing more than being connected to someone who is clicked into autopilot and blind to their acquiescence within a distorted dynamic. This can be tricky if you have people-pleasing or peacekeeping tendencies because the part of you that hopes to be perceived as friendly, accommodating, and easygoing can interfere with what is truly healthy for you. If you navigate such relational patterns, you might fail to notice the red-flag warnings of a toxic relationship. Before you know it, you'll be so far down the rabbit hole that extricating yourself feels arduous. This happens when your inner narrative drives you to prioritize being perceived as good, easygoing, or friendly above all else.

Everyone has different beliefs, values, and priorities, and healthy relationships leave room for individual differences on these fronts. Toxic dynamics, however, tend to be coercive in their efforts to drag you into their perception. People like this want you to see things the way they do, align with their worldview, and abandon personal qualities that uphold the lens of reality that threatens the toxic person's power. Many predatory people possess a disturbing form of calculating, manipulative intelligence that is adept at compelling and controlling you. They know how to put a rosy glow around their opinions and perspectives that's almost contagious as it rubs off on you.

When you're caught in the grip of the "buy-in" trap, your friends and loved ones might mention that you seem different, unlike yourself, when you're around the toxic person. They may express worried feelings and wonder why you have changed your mind on topics you previously felt strongly about. You may also notice that you present in opposition to your true Self, are easily influenced, or often find yourself clouded by confusion when in the presence of this person.

The familiar truism "misery loves company" is similar to what happens with the "buy-in" trap, but it's not always an obvious form of misery. Instead, we can say "toxic people love company." They want you to walk their walk, talk their talk, and believe their beliefs. Why? Because this makes you easier to control and enhances their chances of getting what they want from you— be it narcissistic supply,[1] social reinforcement, or a distorted form of connection where they get to call the shots.

Dynamics like these may seem like no big deal at first, but abandoning your autonomy catches up with you over time. It builds resentment because you disregard your independence, and all that makes you You, in order to cooperate in a relationship with someone who belittles your need for sovereignty and uses you as a means to meet their ends.

Disentangling from the grip of the "buy-in" trap: Cultivate autonomy, explore toxic patterns, identify how you stray from integrity, and develop your personal beliefs and values.

Depending on the relationship, you may notice that you have been stuck in the grip of the "buy-in" trap for a short or long period of time. Sometimes it's not until adulthood that a child of dysfunctional parents gains the strength and self-honesty to recognize this trap. In other cases, lengthy marriages or friendships dissolve when one person chooses to no longer buy into the unhealthy beliefs and values that have necessitated compliance in order to earn love and belonging. In best-case scenarios, a person will notice themselves getting hooked into the landslide of coercion and manipulation early on in a relationship and gently disentangle from this trap.

The most necessary skill when it comes to breaking free from the "buy-in" trap is cultivating the inner autonomy to know yourself and what you believe in without the toxic person's influence. Someone who knows who they are, lives in accordance with their values, and prioritizes integrity is very challenging to manipulate. If a toxic person senses that you are healthy in this way, they may instinctively leave you alone because your integrity immunizes you against their ploys for power and control. If you are a survivor of early autonomy-related trauma and are confused about your right to sovereignty, you may require therapy or other introspective coaching to heal the wounds that block you from such strength. Much of the time, integrity and a values-driven life do not come naturally. These must be consciously cultivated with intentional inner work. After all, you must be willing to gaze inward and attend to the unhealed parts of yourself if you are to sidestep the seductive trap of a toxic person's snares.

Avoid repeatedly getting hooked by the "buy-in" trap in the future: Remain clear with yourself (and others if they are willing to listen) about your beliefs and values, and live aligned with your integrity.

Aligned community, therapy, and other self-reflective practices will help you develop integrity and gain clarity about which beliefs and values are most important to you. As you navigate this work, consider that *beliefs* are the truths you perceive to be most accurate about yourself and your world, and *values* reflect the things, people, and experiences you care most about. When you heal trauma and cease dysfunctional relational patterns, you will naturally steer clear of the "buy-in" trap because you will not be searching aimlessly for connection and belonging at any cost. You will learn to connect with others with authentic integrity,[2] feeling both the *realness* and the *truth* of the bond you share without shape-shifting and self-abandoning to align with a person who dishonors your autonomy.

Once you understand your own value system, you can clearly communicate to others where you stand and more consistently live in accordance with what matters to you. You will also be less likely to collapse into compliant, people-pleasing behaviors because you will recognize this trap sooner and feel more capable of nipping it in the bud. You will no longer invest in transactional relationships that require your buy-in in exchange for connection.

Trap #2: Comfort

The jaws of the "comfort" trap in action: Prioritizing the comfort of others over your own mental health and well-being.

Comfort is the antidote to progress because it keeps you stuck in outdated, possibly unhealthy dynamics with others. For many, the safety of the known present is more appealing than the possible risk of an unknown future born from change. Although the misalignment (or toxicity) of an unhealthy dynamic might not be ideal, at least it's comfortable, right? Wrong.

When you remain stuck in a relationship that is comfortably numb (thanks for the term, Pink Floyd),[3] the true Self within you goes dormant. You lose touch with joy, your capacity for inspiration, and your drive toward meaning and purpose. When these core elements of your true Self get derailed, resentment builds. It may take time for you to notice the irritability, resignedness, and frustration connected to the flavor of resentment that forms when you self-abandon, but eventually it will combust. Resentment is the alert that arises from deep within that screams, *Something's wrong! Redirect course!* It is a sign that you have drifted too far from the essential Self you were born to be, and your inner system has started to revolt.

Change is hard. It requires effort, intention, and resources. This is why it is often easier to remain unhappily comfortable in a relationship that doesn't serve you. For many people in circumstances like this, change activates only when they reach an intolerable unhappiness or a complete lack of safety—and even then, as many in the abuse cycle can attest to, breaking out of a familiar and predictable relationship requires immense strength.

Disentangle from the grip of the "comfort" trap: Learn about how to regulate your nervous system and get to know the parts of yourself that are involved in perpetuating unhealthy relational patterns.

Human beings choose comfort over courage[4] for many reasons, but one of the most common is living from a dysregulated nervous system due to unhealed trauma. When you live and relate from wounds that perpetuate survival mode, you are more likely to make choices that ensure comfort rather than activate growth.[5] This is because your nervous system is wired for survival, not happiness. If remaining frozen or fawning, yet in a predictable circumstance, seems like the surest way to stay safe, that's what your nervous system will do. This is why intentional focus on nervous system regulation is necessary to heal patterns related to intrinsic defaults that have wired *safety* together with *comfort*.

"Parts work" through an Internal Family Systems[6] lens is helpful for healing and rewiring such pathways because it introduces you to the parts of yourself that revert to unhealthy dynamics in an attempt to keep you safe. The part of you that chooses *comfort* is an adaptive mechanism of your inner system. Somewhere in time, this part learned through experience that the discomfort brought on by the risk of initiating change isn't always worth it. Maybe a younger version of yourself got brave, made a major life decision, sacrificed comfort for the risk of a better future, and landed in a heap of trouble. This is how inner safety mechanisms get built upon past experiences in an attempt to predict future safety. Despite the remarkable intelligence of your inner system, sticking with the familiar isn't always a good plan. Why? Because you've come a long way since that early experience shaped your perspective of how to stay safe in an often unpredictable life. You are no longer the young, vulnerable child you were when you built that worldview. You have since grown and evolved into a capable adult who can navigate greater complexity and tolerate disappointment and pain in entirely different ways than your child Self could. Because of this, it is a faulty plan to stick with the fears and blocks your wounded parts insist you abide by. The work of Internal Family Systems therapy teaches you how to unburden and reintegrate the parts of yourself that may be harboring outdated fear and pain so that you can step solidly into the healthiest version of your true Self. We will discuss parts work in more detail in chapter 8.

Avoid repeatedly getting hooked by the "comfort" trap in the future: Relate to others from a regulated nervous system where you can connect with authentic vulnerability and honesty, and reintegrate wounded parts of yourself so that you can connect from your true Self.

If you explore and heal what keeps you stuck in the "comfort" trap of toxic relationships, you will be more likely to avoid getting stuck there in the future. Certain personality types are more liable to get ensnared by the "comfort" trap. If this is you, say "I" and pay extra attention when you feel the seductive pull to settle into familiarity and predictability. You know who you are. Challenge yourself to inquire about the state of your nervous system: Are you feeling activated or numb? Do you notice yourself fawning—responding to others in ways you think will make them happy—rather than standing up for yourself or initiating change in a dynamic? Also notice if there is a part of you that wants to cling to things, people, and experiences that feel comfortable. If you have practiced IFS parts work, you may choose to dialogue with this part of yourself and ask what it fears, what it is protecting you from. With greater awareness, and by consciously cultivating courage and bravery, you can step out of the "comfort" trap and into a bright future brimming with hope, possibility, and healthy behaviors.

Trap #3: Powerlessness

The jaws of the "powerlessness" trap in action: Surrendering power by allowing yourself to be manipulated, gaslit, and abused.

When I write "allowing yourself to be manipulated, gaslit, and abused," I intend no blame or accusation. I explain the "powerlessness" trap with those words to invite you into greater accountability for the role you play in your own powerlessness. The "powerlessness" trap usually involves a person allowing themselves to be made small, insignificant, and easy to control and dominate for the sake of either remaining safe or keeping the peace in a relationship (often both). The first step of healing the "powerlessness" trap is to activate radical Self-honesty that closely inquires about how you have allowed yourself to be dwarfed in relational dynamics.

Powerlessness insinuates victimhood, and it is very possible that you have been victimized by a toxic person. You may have been used, abused, and mistreated in small or large ways. If this is you, please know that I support and honor the wounded parts of you, and I wish only healing for them. Also understand that you will not find healing at the feet of those who currently hurt you. Nor does repair resemble anyone who has brought harm to you in the past. As you are a capable adult, your healing is in your own hands. This is an entirely different reality from what you may have experienced as a young child, chaotic teen, or untethered young adult. It is no mistake that you found your way to this book, this resource for accountability, integrity, and inner work. Some part of you—likely your true Self—is ready to grasp the reins of your life and steer you away from powerlessness and toward empowerment.

If you were made to feel powerless by a toxic person, it is likely that they weaponized your tender heart against you. They may have convinced you that you require their leadership, control, or permission. You do not. Healthy relationships thrive when participants own their power while not seeking to acquire anyone else's power for supremacy or authority. One distorted mechanism of a toxic person is that they often believe there cannot be two strong people in the same room (or relationship). If they sense your strength, they will aim to diminish it to create the contrast where they feel large in comparison to the smallness they have molded into you. This is not love. This is not partnership. This is abusive, manipulative, disempowering, and undoubtedly toxic.

Disentangle from the grip of the "powerlessness" trap: Take accountability for the role you play in your own powerlessness, set boundaries, and do the work to heal your trauma.

The first step toward reclaiming your power is acknowledging that you have participated in surrendering it in the first place. Knowingly or unknowingly, you handed your sovereignty over to a toxic person because you sensed that it was required of you. Perhaps this is the only way you have ever known relationships to be: dominating and controlling. If you wish to regain the power that is your true birthright, it may be the fight of your life—especially if you are retrieving it from a dominant person who has held great influence over you. You may also be battling against the force of multigenerational trauma and ancestral wounds that have perpetuated throughout your lineage for decades (or even centuries).[7]

You must remember that your voice matters. Your personal power is what makes you You, the driving force within that guides your life. You are allowed to have opinions, your dreams are your own, and you can think for yourself. Begin to explore what it feels like to speak up about something you feel strongly about. Notice which boundaries you need to assert and whether they are verbal, nonverbal, delicate, or forceful. You may also need to maintain strong boundaries with yourself that keep you mindful of certain values and healthy behaviors you have repeatedly violated.[8] Play with different expressions of your needs and consider where they might be met most healthfully.

Support is essential as you disentangle yourself from the "powerlessness" trap. Be sure to surround yourself with loved ones who empower your personal agency, autonomy, and free-dom. If you don't have any safe relationships, that is important to recognize. Take the opportunity to build them by seeking aligned people in interest groups, therapeutic communities, or spiritual gathering places. Bring on board a therapist who can help you heal your trauma and understand how you habitually fall into relational patterns that snuff out your voice. When you are surrounded by others who reflect your worth and value, it reminds you of your strength and fortifies your resolve to take back what is rightfully yours—your personal power.

Certain toxic relationships will not survive your empower-ment because they were built on the foundation of your small-ness and powerlessness. As you set boundaries, refuse to engage in dysfunctional patterns, and distance yourself from harmful others, you will likely get pushback as toxic people grasp to re-gain control over you. This is your opportunity to double down and not collapse. It may feel tempting to give in. You may feel emotions like guilt or shame. But you must persevere. A toxic person will eventually move on once they recognize that they cannot fulfill their dysfunctional needs through you. They will skulk away (possibly in a huff-puff of anger, blame, and denial) and find someone else to meet the needs they refuse to heal within themselves.

Avoid repeatedly getting hooked by the "powerlessness" trap in the future: Recognize familiar patterns that insinuate toxicity related to power and control, and steer away from relationships that require your self-abandonment.

Once you know how it feels to be connected to a person who is invested in your smallness for the purpose of their power and control, you will likely recognize this toxicity in others. You may feel more sensitive toward others who diminish your experience, shame you for speaking your truth, or judge you for displaying authentic self-expression. These and many other toxic behaviors indicate that you are not being held within a heathy, reciprocal bond.

The key to avoiding the "powerlessness" trap is to catch it early. Notice if a person demands your self-abandonment before they offer you belonging. If they squash your creativity, shut down your opinions, or shame you for thinking differently than they do, it's a sign that they prefer you to be silent, compliant, and powerless. You may choose to stand against this injustice by communicating your unwillingness to follow their rules for the relationship, or you can simply move away from them. With toxic people, the most effective trajectory is usually the one that involves distancing yourself without necessarily achieving closure or understanding on their part. In most cases, they will not have the capacity to comprehend why you choose not to connect with them because they are never thinking of you in the first place. It is always about them, centered around their need for power and control.

It's okay to protect yourself in any way you feel is necessary. Even going completely no-contact or estranging yourself from toxic family or long-standing friends can be a very healthy choice when you find yourself stuck in a "powerlessness" trap. It's never okay for a person to chip away at your self-worth and constrain your freedom rather than making the effort to recalibrate and balance the dynamic.

Trap #4: False Ownership

The jaws of the "false ownership" trap in action: Considering yourself to be "the problem" and allowing all blame for the relationship's issues to fall on you as the scapegoat.

Let's be honest about one thing: You can't *always* be the problem. It can't *always* be your fault. If you're familiar with this narrative, you are likely the scapegoat for a family or system that benefits from projecting their blame and accusation onto you as a means to avoid owning it themselves. Especially if you stand out from other family members in a certain way—maybe you are somehow different, more vulnerable or sensitive—you may be pegged with the dysfunctional role of receiving the system's shadow projections. This doesn't mean that you are wrong, bad, or "the problem," as you may have grown to believe. Instead, it highlights that there is an issue within the system you are a part of that perpetuates harmful imbalance by placing you in this role.

In some situations, the scapegoat learns that it's easier to just take ownership of the wrong/bad collective material and either handle it all themselves (the "over-functioner") or melt into a puddle of self-hatred and victimization (the "problem child"). In other cases, a scapegoat becomes combative and antagonistic under the weight of the heavy load they have been assigned to carry. Just as imbalance contributes to illness in the body, it also creates toxic, dysfunctional relationships and families that require immense change if they are to achieve healing.

Disentangle from the grip of the "false ownership" trap: Discern the edges between what is yours to own and what is not your responsibility. Begin holding others accountable for their harmful behaviors and dysfunction. Notice parts of yourself that want to heal, rescue, or save others from the discomfort of accountability and responsibility that is theirs to own.

The first aspect of healing as a scapegoat is recognizing the dynamics at play that pegged you in that role. Once you stop believing that you are wrong, bad, or "the problem," you begin to see the system's larger dysfunction. You come to recognize how you have played into the dynamics that cause your suffering and begin to heal through therapy or other self-reflective processes. If others in your system refuse to acknowledge the imbalance and unhealthy patterns of the dynamic, you must gain comfort with allowing them to live in the reality they have chosen. Not everyone will heal. Not everyone wishes to reflect inwardly and take responsibility for themselves. Sadly, a system that has identified a scapegoat has likely grown comfy-cozy projecting their shadow material onto what Brené Brown calls a "common enemy."[9] As Brown says, few things in the world are as fortifying as joining together against someone multiple people have agreed is "bad" or "wrong."

If you have become the common enemy of a system, be it a family, friend group, or professional network, the healing path requires surrounding yourself with healthy people. This might require that you make new connections with people who recognize your gifts and do not shove you into the scapegoat role. Seeking aligned connection in two-person relationships, groups, and communities is essential for the health and mind-body-heart safety that come with true belonging, attunement, and intimacy.

When you take honest ownership of your own unhealed wounds, but not those of others, you achieve a certain kind of freedom that releases you from unhealthy roles. People-pleasing, codependency, and accepting the role of scapegoat can all fall away when you realize that other people's resistance to the inner work that would result in their healing is not your responsibility.

Avoid repeatedly getting hooked by the "false ownership" trap in the future: Courageously take accountability for the issues that are yours to heal, and do not impulsively leap to manage the emotions or experiences of others.

Gabor Mate[10] writes in depth about the healing that is required for the toxic undercurrents in our world. We presently live in a paradigm where unfathomable toxicity exists individually, within families, in workplaces, socially, and even globally. But that's not all. We also live in an era when more people than ever are awakening to wonder if there might be a better way. The ripple effect of either transforming or leaving harmful relationships, unhealthy office environments, and dysfunctional families is spreading rapidly. This the juncture of knowing when to *mend* and when to *move on*. Your participation enhances this powerful movement by contributing to new, healthy awareness and improving expectations for relationships of all kinds.

By engaging your own inner work, releasing the responsibility to fulfill the scapegoat role for others who refuse to look in the mirror, and choosing healthy relationships that align with the highest good for all, you contribute to incredible change. As you walk this path, tread gently and cradle your heart. If you notice the impulse to rescue others from the demons that are theirs to heal, meet yourself with compassion. When you feel the pull to return to old patterns that harmed you, place your hand over your heart and remember your commitment to this work—it's a process that takes practice.

Trap #5: Unhealed Trauma

The jaws of the "unhealed trauma" trap in action: Allowing inner wounds to fuel the repetition of destructive patterns in one (or many) relationships.

Trauma is a bit like a garden weed in the sense that if it is not attended to, it will pop up everywhere—in all the problematic

places, at all the inconvenient times. Your nervous system constantly scans for danger. In fact, this vigilant part of your
anatomy scans your body and surrounding environment four
times per second to discern if you are safe.[11] When something
happens to derail that safety, be it a false alarm or a full-blown
tragedy, your nervous system stores the experience for future
reference so that you have a better chance of protecting yourself against such a threat if it should repeat in the future.

When it comes to relational trauma, your nervous system always seeks safety and tries to repair unhealthy patterns so it
can return to a stable baseline. As altruistic as this may sound,
it often results in the repetition of dysfunction and trauma in
various different relationships in an effort to understand and
work out an issue. After a while, your system can adjust to the
increased threshold that is required to adapt to trauma, so relational hardship can start to feel standard, familiar, even comfortable. You may unconsciously seek out relationships that
mimic familiar patterns because they have come to be normal
for you. This is why the daughter of an emotionally unavailable
father may wind up with a partner with workaholic tendencies
who is unable to be fully present and available for her. It's also
why a person may notice that they tend to fall into repetitive
patterns in friendships or partnerships where traits like narcissism, emotional immaturity, or codependency play out.

*Disentangle from the grip of the "unhealed trauma" trap: Explore
your brain and nervous system's protective neurological wiring. Get
clear on the people and experiences that repeatedly cause harm and
bring trauma into your life.*

The only way I am aware of to disentangle from the "unhealed trauma" trap is to . . . you guessed it . . . heal your trauma.
Sorry, folks, there is no easy button. Intentional work and care

are required, and there's no other way. You must dial into your nervous system, inquire about your wounds, and reflect on your life experiences. Please seek help while you navigate this process—ideally with a clinically trained and professionally licensed therapist, because the going can get rough when you really dig in. A skillful clinician will know how to hold a safe space for your healing in an objective yet compassionate way that will facilitate your deep exploration and repair.

Later in the book you will learn about my personal favorite guide to nervous system healing, which is Steven Porges's *polyvagal theory*.[12] This theory identifies the cranial vagus nerve and its link with the calming parasympathetic function of your nervous system. You will gain both information about and active participation in the health of your nervous system once you gain awareness of how much time you spend in the escalated *sympathetic* (anxious, elevated nervous system state), decompressed *dorsal vagal* (heavy, lethargic, depressed nervous system state), or regulated *ventral vagal* (grounded, calm-yet-energized nervous system state).

In addition to increasing your knowledge of nervous system regulation, many trauma healing modalities are available to you, from EMDR (eye movement desensitization and reprocessing) to somatic experiencing, art therapy to dialectical behavior therapy, Internal Family Systems therapy to psychoanalysis, and many more. Do some research to discover the most comfortable starting place to initiate your trauma healing, and interview several therapists to find the best fit for your needs. Therapy can be time consuming and expensive, yes. But it's a worthwhile investment. Your future Self will thank you. I promise.

Avoid repeatedly getting hooked by the "unhealed trauma" trap in the future: Be cognizant of where (and with whom) you allow yourself to be vulnerable and where you place your trust. When trauma occurs, attend to it immediately and thoughtfully.

Once you attend to your unhealed trauma, it is unlikely that you will fall into that same trap in the future due to your increased awareness of the patterns and warning signs you did not recognize before. Your knowledge of nervous system regulation and the skillset you will acquire in therapy will buoy you if and when you encounter future traumatic experiences. You will also have increased awareness of the particular flavor of harmful relationships and personality types you tend to be most vulnerable to, and you will feel more equipped to navigate or avoid them.

In truth, life presents all of us with challenges that throw us into uncharted territory, derailing our experience of safety in our body and in the world. It's not about never encountering trauma or problematic relationships. That's impossible. Instead, it's about knowing how to notice and attend to them when they present. If you remain agile in your awareness, your nervous system will serve as a trustworthy informant that alerts you to danger, guides you toward safety, and supports your health from the inside out.

Trap #6: Avoidance

The jaws of the "avoidance" trap in action: Making excuses, living in denial, and hoping that relationships will improve with time without facing the root problem.

An ostrich doesn't stick its head in the sand because it likes the grainy texture along its feathers. Well, maybe it does. But really, the old cliché of an ostrich burying itself in quiet sandy darkness exemplifies an avoidant behavior that many people utilize to circumnavigate the pain and discomfort of facing the truth. Like an ostrich, when you refuse to acknowledge whatever would be illuminated in the brightness of day—be it a toxic relationship pattern, your growing unease in a connection or experience, or anything else you would rather hide from than accept as truth—it doesn't eliminate the thing (or person). It simply blocks them from your sensory awareness for a while until you begin to run out of air in the sandy underground world of avoidance you constructed for yourself. And trust me, you will eventually run out of air and be forced to face the truth whether you want to or not.

Your inner compass can tolerate avoidance only to a certain extent before it starts to run your life. This sparks secondary emotions like chronic anxiety and deep-seated resentment as a reaction to the fear and avoidance, and it stirs up somatic symptoms in the body like headaches and digestive issues that alert you to the perils of avoiding the truth. At its core, avoidance is really just a profound level of dishonesty between You and Yourself. It may have negative consequences for others, but ultimately you are the one who will be most severely impacted when you refuse to honor reality. Of course you always have free will, so you can choose to live in avoidance until the day you die, but it will demand a price—likely on your relationships and your mental and physical health.

Disentangle from the grip of the "avoidance" trap: Be brave and lean in with radical honesty to the problematic people, experiences, and behaviors in your life. Make changes in accordance with your discoveries about your unhealthy behaviors and how you participate in cocreating toxic dynamics.

Alright, ostrich. Time to pull your head out of the sand and squint into the discomfort of broad daylight. What? You can't hear me because you're so deeply buried in your own "avoidance" trap? Ease yourself up toward the surface and experiment with allowing glimmers of light (and truth) to reach you. It might be scary, but it's unlikely to be as terrifying as you fear. Like so much in life, actual discomfort is rarely as distressing as we anticipate it to be once we muster up the courage to look directly at the problem. And if it does turn out to be utterly horrific? You've got resources for that in the form of therapy, expert professionals you can source for help, supportive loved ones, and the strength of your capable adult inner Self. At least once you pry your eyes open to observe what you have staunchly avoided you will be meeting yourself honestly. A known truth is always preferable to an unknown possibility, worry, or hidden land mine of fear. At least you'll know what you're working with.

Internal Family Systems (IFS) therapy[13] speaks to the difference between your *true Self* (the essence of your being) and your *parts* (the aspects of yourself that fractal off throughout life in adaptation to challenging situations and experiences in the service of protecting you). If avoidance is your jam, it's highly likely that you have an *avoidant part* of yourself that learned at some point in life that doing the ostrich thing keeps you safe—even if only temporarily. Your avoidant part likely does its best to protect you by repeating behaviors that worked in the past (even minutely, if not ineffectively). Your job as you grow and develop throughout adulthood, acquiring new awareness and tools to positively impact your healing, is to unburden your avoidant part by alleviating the pressure for it to single-handedly protect you.

You may have the clarity of memory to pinpoint the origin of your avoidant part at a certain developmental age or life experience (likely from your early years). An example of this might be a memory of when you were in first grade and your parents reprimanded you with shame and punishment when you expressed your vulnerable need for more attention. Instead of learning that honest communication results in openness and care, you learned to avoid your emotional needs and shut down the softness inside yourself. This adaptation kept you in the good graces of your emotionally dysfunctional parents, which was essential when you were young, but it also taught your inner system that avoidance is key in achieving belonging and safety. Whether or not you can identify the origin of a wound that developed an adaptive part, you can still work with the part as it presents in the moment. You don't have to know the whole story about why it exists, though you may come to understand more as you investigate the part and its purpose (therapy with a trained IFS practitioner is great for this). Either way, parts exploration will help you learn that the part in question may be operating from a set of majorly outdated beliefs and narratives that probably no longer apply to you.

Returning from a dominant part to true Self involves inquiring why you have chosen avoidance over truth. As you grow to better understand the wounds of your avoidant part, you can choose to meet the part with IFS's 8 C's of Self Energy and Self-Leadership[14] to help you return to the orientation of Self. The 8 C's are curiosity, compassion, clarity, connectedness, creativity, courage, confidence, and calmness. When you can feel the presence of several (or all) of the C's, you're likely in Self. From Self, you can make grounded decisions about your life and relationships without being flooded by the wounded and potentially chaotic energy of a part.

Avoid repeatedly getting hooked by the "avoidance" trap in the future: When you feel resistance to inquiring honestly about a problem, challenge yourself to face the problem directly rather than avoiding it, resisting it, or placing blocks between yourself and the truth.

The more you unburden your unhealed parts of the emotional loads they carry, the more you will integrate the exquisite wisdom of your inner system. You may discover that although your avoidant part may have taken ostrich behavior to the extreme, when it is unburdened and integrated it serves as a healthy mechanism for keeping obsessive rumination and hyperfocus at bay. When your parts are balanced, each is inherently valuable and essential to your holistic inner system.

You will notice as you heal and integrate different parts of yourself that the hook to fall into old patterns that once rapidly activated is far less intrusive. Although you may still sense the familiarity of a coping mechanism that you once used as a crutch (like the "avoidance" trap), you will be more likely to sidestep the pattern and choose differently. The more often you challenge yourself to make different, healthier decisions in the face of stress and fear, the stronger your neuropathways will become.[15] Your brain will actually rewire itself away from the "avoidance" trap and toward healthier behaviors that will soon become automatic habits with your consistent practice.

Trap #7: Codependency

The jaws of the "codependency" trap in action: Forming codependent bonds with others and believing it is the same as genuine connection and love.

Remember the oil painting metaphor from chapter 1? Let's use colors to explain codependency: If you are *blue* and the person you are in relationship with is *yellow*, the space where you blend together and overlap in your shared relationship becomes *green.* This is not problematic; it's natural and healthy. Part of why we have relationships is to create the beautiful blend in the center of the Venn diagram where you and another overlap. What does become an issue, however, is when you lose track of your *blueness* and/or the other person's *yellowness* and all you can experience of yourself, them, and the entirety of the connection is a big *greenish* blob that lacks definition and contrast. That's codependency—overwhelming greenishness without the presence of your unique colors anywhere to be found.

In his book *The 5 Personality Patterns*, Steven Kessler[16] describes codependency as the *merging pattern*. It happens when you no longer are a person in a dynamic with another person but instead exist in a blended state of uniformity—what nature calls a "symbiotic organism." In this merged state, your feelings of joy and safety in the world are conditional and dependent on the other person—you're not okay if they're not okay, and until they're okay you won't be. Codependency drains you of your autonomy. It removes you from healthy relationships you previously enjoyed, and it builds dysfunctional enmeshment between yourself and another person that perpetuates unhealed relational wounds from your past.

Disentangle from the grip of the "codependency" trap: Explore where you end and another person begins by inquiring about the patterns of enmeshment and merging you participate in. Begin to learn who you are as an autonomous individual with personal power and unique needs.

You have to return to your *blueness* and allow your counterpart their distinct *yellow* nature if you wish to transform codependency. It helps if both parties are willing to engage in self-healing and reflection so you can heal together, but the other person's participation is not necessary for you to repair your own codependent tendencies. It is likely, though, that if you heal the wounds that diverted you toward the "codependency" trap and no longer wish to operate in that same dynamic, a person who is unwilling to do that work will no longer be a match for you, and the relationship will not survive. In large part, healing codependency is a return to Self. It is an attendance to gaping wounds of unhealed trauma and rediscovery of the beliefs, values, and priorities that make you unique. This is powerful work to explore in couples or individual therapy that includes setting sturdy boundaries between yourself and those you tend to blend with so you can both rediscover your independence.

Dr. Lindsay Gibson's work[17] identifies the link between codependency and emotional immaturity in adulthood, which is a culprit in many codependent relationships. Emotional immaturity is when a person's maturity level misaligns with their developmental stage and age. You might be married to a fifty-two-year-old, but they might behave like an egocentric teenager when confronted with a challenging conversation that requires their accountability. Due to trauma and difficult life experiences, including mental illness and being raised by emotionally immature or personality disordered parents, not everyone reaches adulthood on time (or ever). A person who is emotionally immature (and who comes from an emotionally immature family) will lack the capacity to meet you on adult ground and will revert to unhealthy words, actions, and behaviors that stem from their unhealed child and adolescent material. It can be an aha moment when you realize that you have been in a relationship with an emotionally immature person, and it can also be deeply saddening if they refuse to change. Many people with narcissistic traits, deep-seated tendencies toward denial, or difficulty with compassion and attunement are likely to also be emotionally immature.

Avoid repeatedly getting hooked by the "codependency" trap in the future: Notice when a relationship falls into codependent patterns and address the issue as soon as possible. Relate to others from a perspective of Self with healthy nonattachment.

As Dr. Dan Siegel teaches in his MWe work,[18] humans are essential to one another's health, safety, and stability. It is indisputable that we need each other, that we benefit from human connection, and that we can do incredible things together relationally. Additionally, it is important that our connections be healthy and aligned, not based on unhealed inner wounds and codependency that present as merging, emotional immaturity, or any other form of dysfunctional blending between people.

If you came from a relationally dysfunctional family, you may have an intrinsic operating system that perceives unhealthy bonds as normal and magnetizes toward repeating patterns with others that are unhealthy for you and them. In this case, it may take intentional focus and care to both avoid such dynamics and extricate yourself from them when you realize you have cocreated the "codependency" trap. It's okay, you don't have to be perfect—it's not even possible. Therapy and inner exploration can increase your awareness of such patterns and grow your capacity to mitigate unhealthy bonds as soon as they reveal themselves to you. The time for falling asleep at the wheel of an unhealthy relationship and coasting until dawn in the rickety vehicle of codependency is behind you, don't you think?

A certain level of nonattachment is required for truly healthy relationships. This doesn't mean you are uncaring and cold to your closest people. It means you have a clear sense of where you begin and they end, where they begin and you end. You allow what's their responsibility to be theirs without parachuting in to rescue them in a moment of discomfort, and you acknowledge that their journey may differ from yours in what they are meant to learn and experience. You must let go of control, power, and even the desire to see things from a shared perspective for a relationship to be truly healthy. It is when you appreciate your *blueness* while also honoring their *yellowness* and marveling at the lovely *green* you create together that your relationships will thrive and flourish.

There you have it: The *seven traps of toxic relationships* and how they might show up in your life. If you recognize yourself or someone you know reflected in any (or all) of the traps, great! That's important information for growth, healing, and individuation toward a healthier relational paradigm. The *seven traps* are not death sentences. They do not mean you're doomed and will never find clean, healthy love and belonging. They simply highlight where you might get stuck along the way. When you understand what your hang-ups are, where your wounds are located, and to whom your special flavor of dysfunction attracts you, you come to know yourself better. Discovering new inner depths helps you foster unbelievable healing while breaking free from any bindings that keep you small and unhappy in your connections.

Remember, life is about learning. Just like there are relational traps you can fall into, there is also a rainbow of possibility for the bonds you can build beyond the dysfunction of toxic connections. The next chapter will address the many prospects for how far, wide, deep, and sideways your many relationships might evolve.

CHAPTER 4

The Rainbow of Relationships

Some relationships must end while others need loving nurturance. Certain dynamics benefit from intensive therapy, and others need a firm confrontational conversation. We will explore the infinite array of connections and how they serve you (or don't serve you), but first I want to share a favorite relationship story, as told by Tara Brach.[1]

There was once a couple who had been married for sixty years. They were very open and had no secrets, except for one. The wife kept a shoebox in the closet and asked her husband to never open it or ask about it. Her husband agreed and forgot about the box over time. Years later when his wife became ill, the husband found the shoebox while sorting through her things to help get her affairs in order. The husband took the shoebox to his wife's bedside and asked if they could go through it together, and she agreed. When the husband opened the box, he found $95,000 and two crocheted dolls. Confused, he asked his wife what the contents of the box meant. The wife explained that her grandmother had taught her that the secret to a happy marriage was to never argue. Per her grandmother's teaching, she was to crochet a doll whenever she got angry. This creative act would channel her anger into craft and not toward the relationship. The husband was deeply touched that after sixty years there were only two dolls in the box. This must have meant that his wife had been angry only twice in their marriage! He exclaimed that he now understood the dolls but still wondered about the $95,000. The wife then explained that the money was the earnings she had accrued from selling all the dolls.

So you see, each relationship has its own capacity for the rhythm and grace required to maintain and sustain the peaceful flow of our essential connections. Relationships are not one-size-fits-all, and I'll explain why this is a gift. Imagine the impossible juggle that would ensue if you aimed to pour your heart into all of your relationships equally. You would rapidly find yourself depleted and burned-out to a crisp. Rather, the divine order in the shakeout of relationships is that they come in many shapes and sizes, with differing functions, for short and long durations, in varying intensities, and with wildly diverse embedded invitations for your growth and benefit. Even within a specific category of relationships, like *friends*, there is a broad spectrum. Consider the differences between friends you cherish most intimately and those you enjoy over a cocktail or at a Superbowl party. If you consider the people who have assumed the role of *partner* or *spouse* for you, they likely take on different qualities and degrees of purpose depending on your needs at the time you are paired with them.

It is important to understand that the iterations of relationships are as infinite as a quantum map of timelines in their role and service to your life. This perspective greatly enhances your ability to acknowledge each dynamic—no matter how trying, tumultuous, or traumatic—as grounds for your inner growth, healing, and personal progression.

I always enjoy when books offer the etymology of a word and trace its original meaning centuries back in time for my intellectual pleasure. That being said, I looked up the etymology for the word "relationship" and found it sorely lacking, so I won't offer it to you. Instead, I invented my own etymology(ish) based on nothing historical and from no ancient languages. I like to think of the word "relationship" this way: relation + ship.

> *Relation*: A meaningful connection or knowing between people.

> *Ship*: A vessel that keeps its passengers safe and afloat.

My etymology(ish) highlights our commitment to sail the seas of life in tandem with each other. When we pursue a relationship—a romantic partnership, the intentional conception of a baby, or a pickleball teammate—we begin a type of voyage that no longer consists of only *me* as a singular untethered being. On some level, conscious or unconscious, we make an agreement with another person to do something together—to sail the seas, brave the storms, and navigate the tides to varying degrees dependent on the quality of the connection.

When you consider sailing together, you might visualize a golden sun setting behind a calm oceanic horizon. Conversely, you might imagine a fifty-knot gale keeling an unsuspecting ship to its demise. The truth of relationships is that both extremes are possible, as are the rainbow of prospects between their polarities. So why, then, if a sinking ship is possible, would each and every human being on this floating blue/green planet hop on board? Because relationships are as essential to our physical, emotional, and psychological well-being and survival as breath is to our lungs.

> **How-To Tip**   Visualize or draw an image (or, if you're into writing, write a description) of one relationship from your life represented by a ship (a relation-ship). Use metaphor to represent through imagery or written words the qualities of that relationship. For example, consider if the skies are sunny or stormy (the background quality of the relationship). Perhaps the seas are raging or calm (representing the current situation

the relationship is facing). Notice if the ship's deck seems sturdy or shaky (the foundation of the relationship). Sense whether the ship's sails are in good condition or disrepair (the prospective forward motion of the relationship). Think of other metaphors you can use to represent the quality, stability, and connection of the relationship at hand.

Given that you are reading this book, let's safely assume that you have sailed a fair amount of relationship voyages and acquired some existential questions about the function of your connections and their tendency to cause suffering. Maybe your vessels have crash-landed in a heaping broken mess, or maybe you feel stuck on an expedition you long to escape from within a dynamic that is no longer (or, you realize, possibly never was) healthy for you. If rainbows and hearts are not the exclusive point of relationships (much to the disappointment of our notebook-doodling inner teenagers), then what is?

The Three Types of Relationships

Let's start with the three types. Remember, this goes for all kinds of relationships, so open your mind to consider your favorite waitress, your spouse, your children, your friends, and everyone else in your orbit. Every connection falls somewhere in the camps of *utility*, *pleasure*, and *appreciation*.[2] Each category has room for differing qualities and functions, but they are the three main buckets.

Relationships of *utility* are the those in your life that are the most transactional. They do something you need them to do, and potentially you return the favor. Your favorite waitress is an example of a relationship of utility. She offers you a fantastic dining experience, and in return you pay a large tip and recommend her restaurant to your friends. The utility inherent in service-oriented connections is the easiest to recognize in this category because of the emotional superficiality of such dynamics, but they are not the only type of transactional relationships. Less tangible, more nuanced transactions can also transpire within relationships of utility that affect greater emotional depth.

Patty is a client of mine who struggles to find partnerships where she feels appreciated and honored. She repeatedly finds herself in romantic dynamics with men that begin intensely passionate and sexual before quickly diminishing to rapid endings or painful ghosting. Many deep conversations about Patty's self-worth and early conditioning have helped her recognize that her relational patterns activate a familiar transaction: Patty offers her body sexually (and in other ways) in exchange for feeling loved and desired. The difficult truth Patty has learned is that by participating in relationships that serve this function of utility, she never feels truly loved and appreciated. When she leads with sensuality, she attracts partners who seek sexual ease and its subsequent pleasures before all else. The instant gratification stemming from her promiscuity prioritizes physical connection at the expense of a slower (but more sustainable) relationship built from the joy of each other's minds, hearts, and shared interests.

Certain relationships of utility are healthy and necessary. Imagine the chaos and disorganization that would arise if service-oriented relationships ceased to exist. The key to healthy relationships of utility is having clear, honest expectations of the transaction. It must be mutually understood that your friendly neighborhood mail person's function in your life is to deliver your bills and catalogs, not to join your emotional conversations about childhood wounds or toxic office culture. When the wires get crossed and blending of this sort happens, imbalanced dynamics take root that sooner or later burden, corrode, or explode the connection.

The second type of relationship is one of *pleasure*. These dynamics feel good and bring joy and fulfillment to your life, though they often lack depth and emotional intimacy. Relationships of pleasure connect you to people with whom you enjoy partying, skiing, or catching a spontaneous matinee. In the healthiest iteration of this type, pleasure runs both ways, and each person feels beneficial sparks when they are with the other.

Relationships of pleasure get sticky when they venture toward greater intimacy, responsibility, or intensity than they were built for. Imagine having a fun-loving connection with a coworker built upon company happy hours and occasional weekend brunch dates. Then imagine that it suddenly dives into romantic territory that requires more emotional bandwidth. You are now situated to be a consistent romantic support person and stepparent for three children of divorce when you initially signed up for a casual connection. This is troublesome if both parties don't consent to the shift with their eyes wide open. You're not a bad person if you want nothing to do with the increased intimacy and expectations of diving headfirst into your partner's shifting familial dynamics. Instead, you are a participant in a relationship of pleasure who resists transforming the relationship into a deeper connection of appreciation. And that's okay. The sooner you recognize that your relationship has moved into misalignment, the sooner you can make the judgment call about whether you are on board for the shift or not. Similar to relationships of utility, if relationships of pleasure are respected for their lightheartedness and are not pressed beyond that understanding, they can be a sweet source of joy for both parties.

The third (and last) type of relationship is one of *appreciation*. Ideally, these are your personal and professional partnerships, spousal relationships, closest family relationships, and very best friendships. In a relationship of appreciation, you feel emotionally intimate, trusting, and safe with the other person. Your life is significantly improved because they are in it, as is theirs. You contribute meaningfully to each other's authentic experiences in life, and you show up supportively for one another. These relationships require the most time, effort, energy, and intention, and they also provide the most significant fulfillment.

Relationships of appreciation get sticky when one participant embodies an appreciation mindset and the other person holds one of either pleasure or utility. It is essential for relationships of appreciation to be reciprocal and balanced, or wounding and resentment can occur. Warning signs of an imbalance are feelings of one-sidedness, disregard for each other's emotional experience, and obligation or resentment, to name a few. We will take a closer look at these warning signs, and others, in the section about aligned relationships.

It's worth mentioning that it is possible for each of the three relationship types to transform from one type into another. And there is no perfect recipe where certain relationship types last and others are doomed to failure. Dynamics within all three categories can either thrive or take a nosedive toward a necessary ending. A relationship of utility or pleasure can certainly progress toward the intimacy and commitment of a relationship of appreciation if both parties are on board and conscious of the shift. We attract the relationships we are emotionally ready for. This means we can become ready for a dynamic we previously weren't, and it also means we can decide to lighten the relational load and cool the intensity of certain bonds to more lighthearted or transactional levels. The important thing to remember when you are engaged in a relationship that seems to be tipping from one type into another is this: In order for the change to be effective, sustainable, and healthy for all involved, each participant must consciously acknowledge and agree to the new terms.

Brett and Shawna successfully upleveled their friends-with-benefits relationship to an emotionally intimate, committed partnership when they were both ready to make the leap. Conversations were had (both difficult and exciting), behaviors were modified (they stopped sleeping with other people), and actions were taken (they started checking in with each other more regularly and planning intentional time together). With both partners' agreement and consent, Brett and Shawna built a stable relationship of appreciation from one that originally began casually and without any real promise of a future.

> **How-To Tip**   Call to mind one of each type of relationship you have experienced in your life (utility, pleasure, and appreciation). Notice if you tend toward having more of a certain kind and less (or none) of the other types. If you notice an imbalance in the quality of your relationships, write a list of four or five changes you would like to make to bring greater balance into your dynamics.

Now that you understand the three types of relationships, you can see that our connections with others are far more complex than the roses and butterflies of childhood daydreams about Prince Charming and his true love or soul sisters who remain best friends forever. We need our relationships to provide us with practical tactics to meet our needs, outlets for joy and pleasure, the strength that comes with the supportive commitment, and the meaning and purpose we all yearn for. Sometimes the dynamics fuel and fulfill us for a long time—even a lifetime—and other times they are fleeting and must dwindle to a close.

The give-and-take flow in relationships differs depending on each dynamic. You may discover that you have certain patterns where you negotiate relational dynamics like a default setting. Based on your personal story of what it means to be loved and experience belonging, you likely habituate toward closer kinship with certain types of people. We can all more easily accept certain kinds of love and types of relationships based on what our early conditioning taught us. Each is specific to our individual beliefs regarding our perceived needs and self-worth.

Perhaps you feel most desired in relationships with strong, protective, masculine energetics. This dynamic will attract dominant personalities with an aptitude for caregiving through control, protection, and aggression. Conversely, you may feel most loved in relationships that offer softness, compliance, and agreeableness. This preference attracts dynamics that allow you to be alpha with a much more passive and accommodating counterpart.

Every relationship has many possibilities for its fulfillment and expression, ranging from healthy to toxic, depending on the degree of awareness and trauma each participant brings to the table. The strength and dominance of a masculine energetic can be sustained healthfully, as can a passive nature, but only with awareness and self-insight. It is when we operate relationally from an unconscious lens of habituated patterning that we enter the swampy territory of imbalanced connections that can cause unhappiness and distress over time.

Opposites don't always attract in relationships, like the staunch alpha personality pairing with a demure passivist. Sometimes similar personalities see their own likable qualities in another and are thus attracted. Mostly, however, attraction forms between people who are neither opposite nor similar but something in between. Relationships built on a foundation of mutual respect, curiosity, openness, and healthy attraction need not carry parallel views of the world to remain in nourishing balance. Healthy connection leaves room for individual differences between people that can include diverse belief systems, social aptitudes, values, outlooks, and even political affiliations. Relationships that hold space for differing individual qualities allow two people to foster an intimate dance of connection together. It is key to see one another's differences with an open mind and heart and appreciate what makes them unique rather than forcing sameness.

That being said, studies[3] show that *birds of a feather* tend to make healthier long-term relationships than *opposites who attract*. Though diversity adds to the extensive spectrum of possibilities in our partnerships, friendships, and groups, it simplifies things when two people build a relationship on commonalities that help foster connection and identification with one another.

Along the lines of embracing differences comes the interesting possibility of opening up to new perspectives on how we interact. The COVID-19 pandemic introduced society to the possibility that business, relationships, and even milestone events like birthday parties and funerals can be experienced both virtually and in person. Though there is an irreplicable quality inherent in sharing physical space with those you care about, modern technology has introduced mind-baffling possibilities for people to connect through video chat, send rapid and lengthy text communications, and even sync streaming devices to allow for simultaneous movie watching while being physically present in different locations.

Our technological improvements combined with the busy pace of modern life create an interesting case for digital relationships that do not necessitate in-person contact. As with appreciating the similarities and differences within a relationship, it is likely that a middle ground between full digital and all-in-person is fertile ground for healthy relationships. In fact, Adam Grant, organizational psychologist, author, and Wharton professor, has conducted interesting research[4] surrounding the benefit of hybrid models of interaction that allow for both virtual and in-person workplace dynamics.

Relationships exist in innumerable shapes and forms, from digital to local, with varying personality types, in countless degrees of health and function. To hold the most honest perspective of our propensities toward certain relational dynamics, we must acknowledge the infinite rainbow of possible trajectories for the connections we build. Additionally, we must take accountability for the roles we play in creating and sustaining dynamics with others, for better or worse. The next chapter delves into the truth of the deep relational complexity that unfolds as intricate interpersonal dances between people. Depending on what each person brings to the equation, the dynamic will have predicable pitfalls and speed bumps to navigate. Read on.

CHAPTER 5

The Bittersweet Truth

One of my favorite teachings is my *sunny-side/shadow-side* approach to relationships, which highlights their dualistic nature. Like the two sides of a coin, there are at least two sides to every human experience—and the same goes for relationships. My uncle once told me, "There's your truth, there's my truth, and then there's the truth." Experiences and relationships are more spherical than flat, so the perspectives one can hold about these dynamics are vast. This thought exercise simplifies things to the bright and dark elements of a dynamic so you can explore the contrast. The *sunny-side* is the part (or parts) of your relationship that you gladly show to others, the lighter and brighter aspects—for example, your compatibility or the shared interest that makes you a dynamic duo at Frisbee golf. The *shadow-side* is the part (or parts) of your connection that you likely keep private and hidden—the part(s) that bring you discomfort, pain, and suffering. Examples of the *shadow-side* might be your inclination to bicker or your history of infidelity.

My clients James and Kim enjoy attending professional events together. They work for a large corporation, share big stages for public speaking, and travel the world arm in arm for business-related purposes. The *sunny-side* of their relationship is their amazing synergy in the workplace and how they banter and support one another socially and professionally. Every relationship has both a sunny side and a shadow side, and the shadow side of this dynamic duo is their difficulty when the white noise quiets and they find themselves at home with their two small children. Both James and Kim report feeling a combination of resentment, boredom, and avoidance in parenting that they feel shame and sadness about. They present a façade of being happy, attuned parents at parent-teacher conferences and birthday parties, but the reality at home is disconnected and cold.

James and Kim exemplify one bittersweet truth: relationships are complex, multifaceted, and not always the perfect and pleasurable. Not only do relationships have bright and shadowy qualities but they also have seasons. It is possible that James and Kim will feel differently toward their children once they grow older and share more interests. It is also possible that a change might shift the parents' work dynamic to allow a new perspective toward parenting. Of all the potentiality that may manifest in the future, the *sunny-side/shadow-side* reveals only what is present in the moment. It is a holistic perspective that honors the intricacy of relational undercurrents and invites you to inquire about them. Once you are willing to recognize and accept the dark corners where your relationships do not work for you, it becomes easier to shine the light of curiosity in those directions for better understanding and repair.

Counter to what you may think, the *shadow-side* offers a rich invitation toward growth. Truthfully, we don't grow when we are comfortable. Although the *sunny-side* may feel enjoyable, it's not where the real work happens. Instead, it's where we find reprieve between the shadows that instigate our profound and necessary evolution. The balance between light and shadow importantly keeps our journey unfolding in a healthy direction. The pain points in our relationships persist as such only when we turn away from the *shadow-side* and pretend it doesn't exist. Many people engage in a type of leapfrogging from one sunny moment to another, conveniently skipping over darkness in the hopes that it will magically dissipate. At their core, they know this is both illogical and improbable; however, the discomfort drives them into an avoidant state where they tell themselves they will deal with the shadows later—but later never seems to come. If avoidance is familiar to you, congratulations! You have just clicked into awareness of a pattern that has kept you stuck and unhappy. If you are ready to investigate the resistance and explore the murky waters you've been dodging, let's venture there together.

Mirrors

Relationships are like mirrors. They reflect back the qualities within yourself that you see embodied in those surrounding you. When you feel attracted to someone, it is because they embody something you enjoy about yourself or want for yourself. Maybe they personify something you desire more of in your life. For example, a person who is all too familiar with grief and sadness might be naturally attracted to a joyful, buoyant personality. Your attraction to this person is much more about you than them. It makes sense, really, because you experience life only through your own perception. Everything you see in the world around you is actually in response to yourself. When you feel negativity toward another person or triggered by them, it is because they reflect something back to you that you find intolerable within yourself.

One of my relational triggers is when I perceive someone as being selfish. It irks me to no end. In reality, I'm not triggered because of their self-serving behavior but because of the challenges I experience with allowing myself to behave selfishly. I was taught from a young age that my needs are irrelevant, and I should bump myself to the back and cater to others first.

Because of this conditioning, I came to believe that I am bad and wrong if I take care of myself before meeting the needs of another. Though I have done a great deal of healing surrounding this core belief, it still pops up in certain relationships and gets my blood boiling. My inner growth has allowed me to notice this pattern more acutely so I can better attend to myself and support the continued repair of my emotional wound, but it wasn't always so smooth.

Seeing ourselves in another is what I like to call the *mirror theory* of relationships. What affronts you about others is upsetting only if it highlights something unresolved or unhealed within yourself—otherwise you would feel neutral about it. I imagine this is what therapist and author Terry Real meant when he wrote "We all marry our unfinished business."[1] It is as if one person unconsciously says to the other, "I see me in you." However much they like or dislike what they see determines how they will relate to and perceive their counterpart. Consider it this way: If you met an alien from outer space who behaved in ways you had never before seen or experienced, you wouldn't feel triggered (as long as you felt safe). Instead, you might feel curious. Your awe and wonderment would indicate that you were in the presence of something foreign and unknowable, so you wouldn't project. Rather, you would be available for learning.

We humans tend to share numerous group projections because we are repeatedly and collectively exposed to the same environmental stimuli. We all know love. We all feel hatred and sadness. But there are perceptible differences when you expand your lens beyond the scope of your immediate lifestyle. Culture shock is one example of how we can experience such newness. Different societal customs, beliefs, and living conditions evoke the curiosity and open-mindedness necessary to learn. When you begin to see that dissimilar cultures embrace unique values and lifestyles, it acts as a mirror that reflects the unknown from your perspective. Whether you see uncomfortable reflections of yourself or note your experiential vacancies in another, just remember that humans are immensely valuable walking, talking, breathing mirrors.

Being Needy and Being Needed

I once heard a saying that hit deeply and really stuck with me. It went something like, *you are only as needy as your unmet needs.* Let's be clear about something right up front: Many of your needs must unarguably and unequivocally be met by yourself. Projecting them externally will lead only to disappointment and resentment. For example, expecting another person to validate and uphold your self-worth will never float you for long because this must originate from within in order to truly sustain you. Other needs are appropriate to be met in relationships, such as the need to externally process an experience, co-regulate your nervous system through hugs or other forms of physical touch, and share good news in celebration. It's the process of discerning which is which that often ties people in knots.

A common complaint in many relationships, be they romantic or otherwise, is the push-pull dynamic of *having needs* and *feeling needed.* We all have varying degrees of need we project onto our relationships, so before you start thinking that absolutely no part of you is needy, think again. The real question to consider is how comfortable you are with owning the needs of your inner system. With such awareness you can mindfully ask for certain needs to be met by your loved ones while also taking accountability for other needs you may be projecting that your loved ones are not responsible for satiating. If this sounds like a mind-warp, let me break it down: Certain needs are appropriate for relational fulfillment while others are inner shadows that must be healed internally. We tend to project our wounds onto one another because it initiates a victim-rescuer dynamic that enables us to continually avoid facing our unhealed baggage. When you feel pulled toward external validation or approval, you can be sure you are projecting a need that actually requires inner work to heal.

> **How-To Tip**   Make a few lists that identify your needs and where they can be met most appropriately. If you want to get creative, illustrate your needs as books on a bookshelf. If you have a large need that takes up a lot of space, design your book to be taller, wider, and with a larger spine. Also consider that the book's color reflects the energetic properties of the need (e.g., I consider the color red to be loud and demanding, so I might draw a red book to represent a large, excessive need). If another of your needs is minimal and more in the background, perhaps your book will be gray and narrow. Create a bookshelf for the needs (books) you must meet for yourself, another shelf for those that can be met by loved ones, and another shelf filled with books that represent the needs you are willing to meet for others. Then create a shelf of books that represent needs you have wrongly projected toward inappropriate places (or people).

Francis carried a deep childhood wound in the form of a belief that she is not smart. Her young Self was cruelly reprimanded by an elementary school teacher who told Francis that her brain was slow, and since that time she has strived to prove to the world (but really to herself) that she is smart. About three years into a close friendship, Francis's friend offered the reflection that the know-it-all mindset Francis typically brought into their dynamic was pushing her friend away. Francis consistently shut down her friend's conversational efforts by superseding them with haughty statistics and facts. Her friend simply wanted connection and flowing communication, but the need to feel in-telligent was overriding Francis's ability to access any richness the connection had to offer. Once Francis became aware that her need to feel intelligent had derailed the true connection of her friendship, she committed to healing her inner child's wound so that the friendship no longer served as a battlefield for her unhealed shadow to play out.

Although many needs circle back to inner-child wounds and harmful dynamics in early relationships, healthy needs are cer-tainly appropriate to express within friendships, partnerships, and meaningful connections. In my personal healing journey, I discovered my resistance to admitting that I had any needs whatsoever. I was taught by early caregivers that I could easily be perceived as being *too sensitive* or *too much*. In response to being shut down when I expressed needs for belonging and con-nection, I developed a plan for emotional safety: If I needed nothing from others, I could sidestep their rejection and sim-ply tend to myself without being hurt by anyone. As an adult, I see how this hyper-independent narrative is filled with holes like Swiss cheese. But as a child it seemed like a pretty solid plan.

Throughout my younger years I was an agreeable *good girl* who never let myself need too much. Soon enough my adaptive behaviors leapfrogged into adult relationships where I became the giver who asked for very little (ahem, nothing) in return. Without any needs, I would certainly avoid pain, right? Wrong. This is what happened: Ignoring my needs did not eradicate them. Over time, each of my connection-related yearnings, longings, and requirements spiraled inside like a coil that even-tually could not help but spring outward. I sustained my stoic position as the giver without needs until I couldn't tolerate it anymore, and then the spring broke loose. Resentment for the one-sidedness that had developed consumed me, and because the unhealthy dynamic was foundational to the connection, the relationship ended. This happened in several relationships until I was able to notice and attend to the pattern.

When I reached the point where I could finally have a direct and loving conversation with a close friend about my unmet needs in our relationship, I knew I had grown. Taking accountability for the parts of myself that needed warmth, kindness, consistency, and care allowed me to break the spell I had entranced myself within for so much of my life. This particular friend's ability or inability to pivot in adjustment to my newly expressed needs became irrelevant as I witnessed my healing unfolding.

It is no secret that Western society's narratives about the needs and neediness of people imply an undeniable negativity. However, the feeling of being *clingy* or *needy* is not necessarily a bad thing, though it can be quite uncomfortable for all involved. This is why I like to remember that you are only as needy as your unmet needs. There is no universal measuring stick for how needy is too needy; it is defined within each connection (usually indirectly). Depending on the capacity and tolerance of those involved, as well as the emotional experiences and unhealed wounds they bring into the dynamic, every person's ability to hold space for another's needs—and their own—will differ. When I notice neediness or clinginess within myself, I find it fruitful to gaze inward and question why such feelings arose. In some cases, I may be projecting shadow material that requires inner healing, and in others it is possible that the relationship cannot meet a very reasonable and appropriate need. Either way, when I remove the criticism and judgment that accompany my neediness, I am able to see an undoubtably misaligned relationship that derailed long ago, though I likely neglected to notice it. Only by perceiving the experience as information without emotional attachment can I inquire whether a relationship is repairable or not and take accountability for the aspects of the dynamic that are mine to heal.

The flip side of being the needy one in a relationship is being the person who feels either suffocated or gratified by another person's neediness. If you feel suffocated by and resentful about meeting someone's needs, that's good information about your own interpersonal needs as well as your capacity for others. If you feel deliciously gratified when you fulfill the needs of another, it may indicate that your own needs for caregiving are being met when you take care of others: needing to be needed—another excellent dynamic to be aware of.

In the healthiest sense, a relationship should feel like the rowing of a boat down a stream (remember relation-ship?). Sometimes it requires more paddling on one side than the other to regain balance, but overall the vessel is carried forward by equal partnership. If you notice yourself feeling needy and clingy much of the time, or if you notice yourself resisting or luxuriating in the needs of another, you've got yourself an imbalance. If a boat is paddled too much on one side without enough paddling on the other, it will start circling and lose sight of its course. The same thing happens interpersonally. A great way to notice such an imbalance is to acknowledge and attend to the need dynamics.

> **How-To Tip** If you want to start expressing your needs but you're not sure how, here's a starting place:
>
> 1) Identify within yourself an unmet need. Notice the void within yourself and identify what might fill it. Then discern if your need seems appropriate to be met by a relationship or not.
>
> 2) If you deem your need one that is important to meet for yourself, refrain from projecting and attend to it with

> your inner toolkit or with the support of a licensed therapist. If it is appropriate for your need to be met relationally, express it to your loved one in affirmative language. Try not to speak about what's not working. Paint a picture about what it would look like if your needs were being met flawlessly. Notice the difference between "You don't call me often enough" and "I would really appreciate if you would call me more often."
>
> 3) If the person takes your need seriously and tries to meet it, be sure to express gratitude. Appreciation is encouraging and can motivate your counterpart to continue the new behavior.

If you are unsure about the health and alignment of your relationships, the following three questions will help guide you. Spoiler alert: The answer to all three should be *yes* if you are in alignment, and you should have a clear sense of *why* and *how*.

1. **Is this relationship intentional?** If your relationship is intentional, it means that you have consciously chosen to remain in it day after day. You weren't accidentally thrown together and tied to the mast of your relation-ship by anyone. You have a clear sense of the connection you share with your counterpart, and you decidedly choose them. If you find that your relationship is not intentional, or no longer intentional if it started out with clarity and decisiveness, you may be on an autopilot setting that perpetuates your connection without your consent. When you engage with others from cruise control, you are passive to the dynamic and unclear about the reasons for your bond.

2. **Is this relationship balanced?** Balance is a tricky thing in relationships because it's not always fifty-fifty. Even

the healthiest relationship vacillates in the energy each person funnels into it, but overall, the healthiest relationships are reciprocal. This means that both people feel seen, heard, understood, and valued. Both people feel comfortable asking for their needs to be met and communicating when something feels off. If your relationship is imbalanced, you may feel like you are always the one giving or most often the one who reaches out. You may also feel like you are consistently relinquishing your voice or power so that the other person's voice and power can direct the relation-ship.

3. **Is this relationship serving the highest good of all involved?** Let's be honest, you probably already know if your relationship is serving everyone's highest good or not—you just may not be honest with yourself about what you know. You know? Your gut will tell you if your relationship feels wonky. You will notice resistance in your body when it's time to see that person. Your thoughts might be judgmental and critical. Basically, you won't feel filled up and satisfied by your interaction, and possibly you'll feel their lack of interest or disappointment in you as well. When a relationship is serving everyone's highest good, it feels nourishing. You think highly of one another, speak highly of the other when they are not around, and look forward to connecting with them.

By answering each question honestly in the present moment (because the answer in the past or future might be different depending on oh so many factors), you offer both yourself and the person you are connected to a particular kind of freedom.

When a relationship is intentional, balanced, and serving the highest good of all involved, both parties benefit enormously from the bond. The healthy dynamic contributes to a cascade of positive psychological, emotional, and physical benefits that sustain and nurture multifaceted health for both people. The relationship flows and generates affirmative messages to each person's nervous system that they are safe and valued. If you answer these three questions with a resounding *yes*, congratulations! You've got a healthy dynamic. Your job in this scenario is to meet the other person halfway by continually nourishing the relationship in the specific ways it requires to keep it sailing along buoyantly.

If you landed on the flip side when answering the three questions, discovering that one or more of them is a *no*, don't freak out. We ask honest questions so we can ascertain honest answers and thus open doors for our freedom and growth. If your relationship (or multiple relationships) feels unintentional, imbalanced, and/or not serving the highest good of all involved, I'm glad you decided to face the music. Knowing what is not working in a dynamic is as important as knowing what is (if not more so). When you truthfully discover that you have been limping along, over-functioning, shrouding yourself in denial, or perpetuating avoidance about the misalignment of a relationship, you crack open the door to freedom. All impactful change begins with the observation that something feels funky enough to look closely and consider altering it. If you are now aware that change is necessary in one or more of your dynamics, it's okay if it feels scary at first. With thoughtful consideration and self-honesty, your clarity will continue to unfold.

One of the most bittersweet truths of relationships is that alignment is not consistent throughout time. What once was brilliant and supportive between people may take a nosedive into coldhearted disconnection. What once felt strong and genuine may shift into fragility and inauthenticity. It is not important that relationships last in the emanant glow of their glory forever. It is important that you notice the imbalance of a connection that was once aligned (or perhaps, you realize, never truly was) and make accordant shifts to regain balance. Remaining flexible and willing to pivot is beneficial for your relationship with your Self and also for the sake of others. Altercations that call out a problematic dynamic may feel upsetting or triggering in the moment, but in hindsight most people discover that the misaligned relationships they shifted or released did truly necessitate such measures for their happiness and health.

Speaking of triggers—you may discover that misaligned relationships (and aligned ones too, to some extent) can be triggering in certain ways that predictably curdle your stomach. The next chapter addresses several impactful triggers for your deeper integration and understanding.

CHAPTER 6

A Chapter About
Triggering Words

Sticks and stones may break my bones, but words will never hurt me. Yeah, right. Anyone who was once a child intoning this familiar chant likely knows how difficult it can be to let words slide away like rain down a metal roof when they so often pack a powerful charge. For those among us, myself included, who identify with Gary Chapman's *words of affirmation* love language,[1] you likely understand the power words possess to sculpt relationships—for better or worse. In best-case scenarios, thoughtfully chosen commentary can make someone's day, act as a support net, or foster the healthy foundation for a new relationship to grow. But we do not always use language for the best-case scenario, do we?

Word choices also have the power to destroy relationships by causing fractures between people that can result in breakups and highly charged no-contact scenarios within families. Consider the hurtful comments so many family members make toward one another over seemingly innocent family dinners or the passive-aggressive remarks exchanged between friends at a casual happy hour. In some cases, words transform into weapons that are used to get revenge, wound someone's pride to make them feel small and insignificant, or plant seeds of doubt that threaten to grow into dangerous worry and obsession.

Depending on how you wield them, words can be wildly triggering, deeply hurtful, inquiry-provoking, or loving and profoundly healing. When you take responsibility for the words you use, you harness their impact and become more mindful of using them with care. After all, words are tools—communication tools—and you are given the opportunity to use them in a multitude of ways each and every day. Tremendous satisfaction can be found in the nuance and expression of a triumphant *aha!* feeling when you find the words that seamlessly fit a particular moment's experience. Words potently paint descriptive pictures about your communications and introspections. For better or worse, deep gratification is available when we grab the magical combination of words that highlights joy, expresses deep sorrow, or wields a painful sucker punch to the gut. In this chapter we will explore the potency of seven words that exist within most relationships in some shape or form and can be wildly triggering to even the most unassuming communicators.

1. *Triggered*
2. *Unconditional love*
3. *But*
4. *Happy*
5. *Bored*
6. *Fear*
7. *Emotional immaturity*

When a person gets triggered by a word (or words) it is likely that something upsetting has been unearthed conversationally that negatively reflects their intrinsic worth, behavior, lovability, capacity and bandwidth, or value. This activates their nervous system, which instantaneously spreads a flood of neurochemicals throughout the body to protect the sensitive area that has been hurt, shamed, angered, or humiliated. The speed at which the nervous system responds to a trigger explains why we can react explosively to something that was said to us (or about us) and later recognize our response was an overreaction. We get triggered because we are human. We care how we are perceived, we want to be liked and valued, and it irks us mentally, emotionally, and physically when things go awry in this territory. Inconveniently, our interpersonal interactions bring emotional content that makes us uncomfortable to the surface of our awareness. Because most people feel great discomfort with feeling uncomfortable, we tend to react severely when triggered. We lash out, create drama, shut down, or behave chaotically in an effort to diminish the undesirable emotional experience we would rather not tolerate. Even the words "trigger" and "triggered" are triggering for many people, which is where we will begin our exploration.

Triggered

I am so triggered by what you said. I feel so triggered right now. You always get so triggered when I do/say that.

Familiar? I thought this one might be. Even the word "triggered" is so undeniably triggering, its hashtag has been banned from many popular social media apps. If that's not power, I don't know what is in this modern age. If people get triggered simply by the word "triggered," you can safely assume that much of society is walking around with unhealed material just beneath the surface of their quivering smiles and dodgy eye contact. If a person is consistently triggered in a specific relationship, it can indicate a serious problem in the emotional safety and quality of the connection. Ultimately, we want our nervous systems to be calm and regulated in our relationships, so feeling frequently triggered by someone close to you is a red flag that requires honest reflection. It doesn't necessarily mean that the relationship is doomed to end, but rather that something important needs to heal if the connection is to continue.

I have developed what I call the *wormhole theory of triggers* because integrating scientific vocabulary into the broader human experience is fun. In Christopher Nolan's 2014 blockbuster movie *Interstellar*,[2] a group of astrophysicists and astronauts devised a plan to bridge large distances through space-time travel in order to explore new worlds that could potentially save humankind as we know it. One poignant scene involved a character named Romilly explaining the logistics of galactic wormholes connecting two distant points in space-time by acting as a type of funnel between them. He folded a piece of paper in half to represent consolidating the expansive mass of the universe by allowing opposite sides of the paper to touch (modeling two distant galactic points coming into conceivable proximity). Romilly then poked a hole across both sides of the folded paper to represent a wormhole connecting the two once-distant-but-now-adjacent locations. Voila! Space-time travel through a wormhole.

Now let's connect intergalactic wormhole travel to triggers. When you are caught in a triggering moment, it is as though the entire universe of your skills, tools, and attuned awareness of all things human (all represented by the piece of paper) gets folded in half and is quickly bypassed by the tunnel (i.e., wormhole) that connects the stimulus (whatever triggered you) and your response (an impulsive emotional reaction). In essence, your trigger acts as a teleportation device that catapults you at lightning speed past rational, grounded, realistic, and conscious knowledge that could potentially mitigate a response you might later regret.

In his groundbreaking book *Man's Search for Meaning*,[3] Victor Frankl explained that between stimulus and response there exists a space where we have the power to make choices that can ultimately contribute to our freedom. In short: Don't get hooked into your triggers, bypass your rationality through a wormhole, and react impulsively before you take a nice solid pause for inquiry. When you gift yourself a chance to choose a response that will best serve your highest good, you also offer your nervous system the biological equivalent of a soothing cup of chamomile tea. Once stabilized and regulated, you can relate to whatever triggered you from the battery of tools, curiosities, knowledge, and resources you so conveniently hold within yourself rather than defaulting to an absolute frenzy. In this case, it's best to opt out of the convenient wormhole that quickly whizzes you from *here* to *there* and take the scenic route instead.

> **How-To Tip**   Explore a familiar trigger in your journal, one you feel safe and stable to write about, and consider how you can bypass the wormhole. If you're feeling artsy, make a drawing or painting of the wormhole.

Unconditional Love

My love for you is unconditional. If you loved me unconditionally you would never have done/said that. Unconditional love is the goal.

Let's just get this out of the way up front: Outside of a parent or caregiver's love for their young children, unconditional adult love isn't a real thing. There, I said it. *Unconditional love* has become a buzz-phrase that most often leaves people feeling guilty or shut down for having needs. I'll explain: We all have conditions for our relationships if you dig deeply enough, even if those conditions are as simple as requiring kindness and participation in or commitment to the relationship. These basic relational needs, as well as any others you may have, are not only acceptable, they're essential. Think of someone you think you love unconditionally. Then imagine the deal-breaker—there's always a deal-breaker if you are honest with yourself. Get creative and stretch your mind for a moment to the worst-case scenario. Imagine if this person falsely accused you of a crime that is punishable by life in prison. Visualize how you would feel if they sucked all the kindness and respect out of their treatment of you, leaving you with only hateful bitterness and cruelty from them. Envision them slandering your character to everyone who respects you. Yep, I went there. And you can too. As you call to mind the atrocities of such potential experiences, notice how the unconditional love you feel toward this person shifts. You are now coming face to face with the limits of your love. Unhealthy, dysfunctional relationships will push the limits of your love on a regular basis, and that's how you will know when it's time to *move on*. Conditions are a good thing because they protect you and set the standard for the kind of treatment you are willing to tolerate.

As an example, I'll talk to you about the conditions implicit within my marriage—which I consider to be very healthy, happy, and stable. My husband, Danny, and I have ridden in tandem many of life's waves during our twenty-two years together. We have been gentle with each other during some phases, firm and confrontational in others, and usually sensitive to each other's wants and needs. There's not a lot about Danny that irks me, and we don't follow particular rules you might typically consider *conditional*. Instead, conditions come into play in the way we both expect to be treated. If Danny one day woke up with a personality shift and started treating me with manipulative, controlling, or power-hungry dynamics, it would be a big problem for me. If he had an affair, became abusive, or made unilateral decisions about our shared assets, we'd have a colossal issue. These are some of the limits of my love for Danny.

You may be thinking that these are basic, universal expectations we should all have for healthy relationships, and you're right—but they're still conditions. There is an edge to what I will tolerate, even in my heart-bonded partnership. No matter how committed I am to Danny, I will not allow him to wreak havoc on my heart, mind, soul, or body. And that's why there is no such thing as unconditional love. True unconditionality would operate under the premise that nothing Danny could do, no matter what, could fracture my love for him. If I told you that's how I feel, I would be lying—and so would you if you claimed the same. We all have conditions. Some of them are universally accepted, and others are particular and individualized. It doesn't matter exactly what your conditions are in your relationships; it matters only that you are cognizant of your conditions and conscious of your counterpart's as well. With such knowledge and awareness intact, one person can honor and respect their personal limits and those of another, and healthy relationships can thrive.

Why were we sold the narrative that true love should be unconditional? As you consider this fallacy, remember that humans weren't given claws or warm woolly coats for survival; we were given each other. It is our relational duty to express our needs to one another while also honoring and doing our best to help fulfill the needs of those we care for to the degree that it is healthy for us. That's where it gets tricky where unconditional love is concerned—discerning the tipping point where healthfully expressing and meeting each other's needs crosses over into the territory of codependency, relational abuse, or interpersonal toxicity. These are unhealthy dynamics no matter how thoroughly you attempt to convince yourself of the opposite. Too much dependency on another person and excessive avoidance of loving support can result in the fallacy of unconditional love being the cornerstone of a relationship.

Hear me when I say this: Loving someone without conditions and tolerating abuse or unkindness is not unconditional love. It's a trauma response. You may have picked up such dynamics in your childhood relationships with caregivers or somewhere else along your journey, but please understand that it's not real love if it is tolerant of maltreatment and cruelty. Rather than authentic love, this type of participation in unhealthy dynamics is your nervous system's adaptive mechanism for keeping you safe while under the spell of a narrative that says you must placate and fawn in your relationships to earn belonging, love, and security.

When someone pulls the *unconditional love* card in an argument or charged conversation, it could be wildly triggering for you because it acts as a shutdown mechanism that ends the conversation with a brick wall. You might be neck-deep in a disagreement with your spouse about something you truly care about when out of nowhere they shout, "If you loved me unconditionally you would never ask this of me!" They're triggered and you're triggered. What is there to say in response to a comment like that? It's the red card that gets pulled to put a one-sided hard stop to a conversation where a person won't flex. On the flip side, when someone uses the phrase "unconditional love" in an intimate moment of heartfelt connection, it is a hopeful promise that is impossible to keep. Imagine two lovers in bed, flooded by postcoital streams of oxytocin flowing through their brains and bodies, and one lover says to the other, "I love you unconditionally. There is nothing you could ever do or say that would change that." Sure there is. Revisit the worst-case scenario possibilities explained earlier and see if you still feel the same unconditionality toward any other human being on the planet, no matter how passionate or loving they behave in a heated embrace.

To set yourself up for healthy relational dynamics that have the flexibility necessary to hold space for each person's growth, changes, and inner makeovers throughout life's winding journey, I propose that you consider using the phrase "deep commitment" instead of "unconditional love." Deep commitment honors your heartfelt connection and depth of commitment to another person while allowing space for you to be a continually evolving being of growth and change. My guess is that you don't want your relationships to be like cages. More than likely, you would prefer for them to feel like nests that both safely hold you and allow you to feel free.[4] *Deep commitment* is a healthy container for meaningful relationships that grants space for you to invest your heart without codependency, toxicity, or unhealthy sacrifice.

> **How-To Tip**   Make a list of your relational conditions. Go ahead, it'll be good for you. Remember, you will have different conditions for different kinds of relationships. If you'd like, make a list for each type of relationship. No matter how ordinary or basic your conditions are, consider how important they are to the health of your connections.

But

I hear what you're saying, but I feel differently. I know you want to go to Disneyland, but I don't want to go. I love you, but I can't do that.

If I could, I would vote the word "but" off the island and re-place it with "and" in all cases. The word "but" is most often used in the English language to invalidate a person's feelings or ex-perience or to redirect a conversation away from accountably and toward defensiveness—which is why it is so, so triggering. Dysfunctional relationships often use the word "but" to shunt responsibility for emotional maturity and sensitivity toward one another's needs and experiences. If you're trying to *mend* a meaningful connection that has posed problems, I suggest throwing "but" into the bushes and learning how to use the word "and" instead. With the simple swap of "but" for "and," your problems can be avoided by allowing the dismissive nature of "but" to be replaced by the inclusivity of "and." Notice if you can feel the difference between these two statements:

- I really love you, *but* I can't tolerate it when you yell at me.
- I really love you, *and* I can't tolerate it when you yell at me.

In the first sentence, "but" obliterates the portion about love like an eraser passing over a chalkboard. In the second sentence, "and" allows for love to exist while the expression of feeling is communicated. It allows room for both to be true—the love and the emotion their behavior has ignited.

Using inclusive language by replacing "but" with "and" soothes a person's defensive response to criticism by allowing them to feel seen and valued while also being taught about the harm or discomfort they caused (knowingly or unknowingly). When a person feels that their intentions, value, or very existence is confirmed by inclusive language, they become significantly less likely to respond defensively, aggressively, and with denial. Therein lies the possibility for healthy repair that incorporates the conscious involvement and regulated nervous systems of two people who ultimately aim to peacefully coexist.

You may use the word "but" to unintentionally dodge blame, avoid discomfort, or win an argument. As you become aware of the function this seemingly innocent three-letter word serves for you, see if you can extricate your own resistance to using inclusive language during a moment of conflict in your relationship. You may discover that you are in some way committed to feeling *right* and making the other person *wrong* to confirm your rightness. It is possible that by using the word "but" you avoid feeling the discomfort of acknowledging another person's feelings and genuine experience because you feel resistant (on some level) to understanding their point of view. Maybe your utilization of "but" allows you to maintain the role of martyr, victim, or righteous one that you have unconsciously formed an attachment to. When you begin to understand the *why*, you can get curious about how different your relationships (and subsequently your life) could look if you dropped the "but" and picked up the "and." My guess? You will likely notice more vulnerability and trust within your relationships in response to your inclusivity, humility, accountability, and openness. All that by swapping out one measly three-letter word for another.

> **How-To Tip** Notice how often you use the word "but" and in what contexts. In your journal, write the common phrases you often use the word "but" in, and write alternative phrases that swap out "but" for "and" (like I did in the example). Read them aloud to yourself and notice how different they feel.

Happy

I just want you to be happy. You make me so happy. I am happy we found each other. We used to be so happy together.

Socrates first suggested that happiness is a cognitive meaning-making pursuit. Rather than buying into the previous assumptions of the time—that happiness was a gift from the gods—he believed that human beings are in control of their own happiness. Fifty years after Socrates died, two competing interpretations of his philosophy of happiness emerged from the philosophers Aristotle and Aristippus: *Hedonism* was defined by Aristippus as the type of happiness that comes from pleasure, and *eudaemonism* was identified by Aristotle as the type of happiness derived from meaning and purpose. Aristotle found his colleague Aristippus's development of hedonism to be based on vulgarities he distained, so he developed the concept of eudaemonia with the ideal of "living well" as its definition.[5]

In alignment with the concept of eudaemonic happiness is the work of Shigehiro Oishi from the University of Virginia[6]. Oishi reviewed a year's worth of obituaries and discovered "psychological richness" as one of the measures commonly stated as contributing to a life well lived. Embedded in the fabric of psychological richness was consistent evidence of fascination and wonder, which became known as its hallmarks. In fact, living a wonder-filled experience seems to be a more complete and holistic intention than any singular form of happiness could ever possibly be. Let's face it, wonder embraces the messiness and complexity of life in a way happiness alone simply cannot. And it can be incredibly triggering to be continually pressured to feel happy all the time when it so profoundly lacks the depth of wonder, fascination, awe, and marvel. Some of the unhealthiest relationships overlook the value of emotions like wonder and simply demand perpetual happiness, requiring happiness or nothing. This is problematic because happiness is too general a goal to encompass the nuance inherent in human experience and interpersonal connection. When it comes to happiness in relationships, what matters most is discerning whether on-going fulfillment is possible without forming an attachment to either type of happiness as the be-all and end-all but instead integrating a healthy balance of both.

The English word "happiness" comes from the Icelandic root *happ*, which means luck.[7] This insinuates that luck has something to do with happiness, which I find to be both interesting and quite relieving. In relationships, luck does play a tremendous role. In order to build and sustain a happy relationship, you must first be lucky enough to meet one another, both be in the open-minded state of welcoming a relationship, and happen to have the space, time, and energy to nurture it. That's a lot of luck involved just at the inception and early stages of connection, let alone what is necessary for the long haul. As a relationship progresses, luck remains present in a person's capacity for the qualities that enhance the strength of the bond. One such quality is *sympathetic joy*, which is the phenomenon of taking joy in other people's happiness. The opposite of envy, sympathetic joy nourishes relationships from the inside out because it sidesteps selfishness by holding precious the happiness of another person.

Whether you are considering sympathetic joy, exuberance, contentment, or any other form of happiness, it is truly ironic to consider how prized happiness is in our Western culture of such chronically unhappy people. Here are a few pre-COVID statistics that will get you wondering why any of us should expect happiness as a baseline for our relationships: Globally, 280 million people have a diagnosis of depression. In the United States alone, forty million people have anxiety. Additionally in the United States, $200 billion is spent every year on treating mental illness.[8] That's a lot of evidence that happiness is more elusive than our fantasies might lead us to believe. With such high levels of mental illness and emotional instability, perhaps happiness is too large a goal to be placed on the mantle of our hopes and dreams. First, if we are to be truly happy, we must attend to the root problems within our culture and society that stand as blockades between us and the happiness we so yearn for—both relationally and otherwise.

One culprit that aids in the smoke-and-mirrors fantasy of our quest for healthy, happy relationships is our poor *affective forecasting*. This term describes how we predict we will feel at any point in the future about a given person or situation or even ourselves; it is how we forecast our emotional experience. As it turns out, people are not proficient affective forecasters. We tend to grossly misjudge what will make us happy by attaching our projections for satisfaction on illusory or material ideals such as wealth, popularity, status, Ferraris, and ski chalets in the Swiss Alps. We distract ourselves with material possessions and the acquisition of more fancy fluff to the distraction of what truly fills our cups with happiness: deep interpersonal connection, quality time with both ourselves and our loved ones, creative pursuits, and intentional cultivation of a wonder-filled life in awareness of the tiny sparks of joy and aliveness that make us feel at home within ourselves.

How-To Tip   Write about your barriers to happiness in your journal. Consider where you may be getting in your own way.

Bored

I am bored in this relationship. You bore me. I feel like I bore you. You seem bored.

Psychologists who have studied boredom in both children and adults discovered that some of the most creative, innovative acts and inventions arise out of unstructured (boring) moments when a person allows their mind to simply exist in a low-novelty, low-stimulation moment without intervention. If we let them, moments of boredom act as a type of empty container awaiting filling by some unexpected igniting force. But what about boredom in relationships?

As it turns out, boredom is not what it seems. It is not the uneventful lack of stimuli linked with tediousness, lethargy, and a certain tension-filled experience of restlessness—well, not exclusively, anyway. In actuality, boredom is quite complex and nuanced—and triggering! It can indicate many different interior phenomena and point to a variety of psychological, emotional, or sensory experiences. For example, there is *simple boredom* and *existential boredom*.[9] These terms outline the difference between not having anything to occupy your time while awaiting a train (simple boredom) and feeling an underlying sense of wariness related to lacking purpose on a soul level (existential boredom).

I'll add a concept I call *relational boredom* into the mix, which is the experience of feeling uninspired or uncharmed in connection with another. I perceive relational boredom to be a message from deep within your psyche that something regarding an important interpersonal connection is too uncomfortable to allow yourself to feel, so you unconsciously choose boredom as a means to avoid discomfort. Let's face it, it can be much easier to feel bored than admit to yourself and your spouse that you no longer feel sexual attraction toward them. Or that you are so annoyed by the way they chew their dinner that you're contemplating the possibility of never eating together again. Or that your common interests have devolved to the singular topic of discussing the strange mating behavior of the squirrels who live in your backyard.

When a relationship dynamic has settled into boredom, you can bet boredom isn't the actual problem. It simply masks the actual problem no one really wants to admit to or deal with. This type of awareness is a *Matrix*[10]-style blue-pill-or-red-pill dilemma of sorts: You can keep swallowing the blue pill, which will effectively help you deny any issue in the relationship and keep you comfortably (though really uncomfortably) detached by feeling bored. Or you can chuck the blue pill and kick back the red pill, which will bring you face to face with underlying malfunctions and issues that lie hidden beneath the companionable surface of your seemingly satisfactory relationship. As with Neo, the choice is always yours. But if you keep downing the blue pill, stop saying you're bored and just admit that on some level you are unhappy and unwilling to investigate why or repair the problem.

Boredom is intimately connected to stimuli and novelty or the lack thereof. Occasionally as a form of self-care, my client Joseph whisks himself away from his everyday normalcy of family and real-life responsibilities for a couple of solo days in the mountains. The location he frequents is the bustling base village of a ski resort. Though Joseph enjoys a day of skiing or hiking, there's a special permission he cocoons into on these short escapes from reality. Somehow, in the midst of such a noisy scene, Joseph introverts away into his own space where he feels unpressured to do much of anything, despite everyone else's high energy and mingling. It's a paradoxical experience counter to what you might imagine, but the change of scenery and high stimulation offer Joseph's nervous system the invitation to selectively decline in an experience that's sweet and nourishing for him.

This type of experience, the contrast of high vs. low stimulation, is a swinging door. Sometimes something that feels quite the opposite of Joseph's quiet reverie happens in relationships. Sometimes amid the stable, steady cadence of a long-term adult relationship, people crave the stimulation of drama and activation. They often think of this as a diversion from boredom. It's not necessarily a problem if you observe and answer your system's call for novelty. All humans get restless when they are exposed day in and day out to the same rhythm. It's not about never feeling bored in your life, routine, or relationships. It's about attending to the call for freshness when it arises. This allows you to satisfy the urge in a healthy way so you can return home to the stability and familiarity you have chosen to be your daily existence.

> **How-To Tip**   What is your sensory experience of boredom? What does it feel like when you're bored? Consider your body, mind, and emotions. Maybe you feel exhausted, irritable, or heavy in your heart. Journal about how you could counterbalance that energy and how your efforts might be healthy or unhealthy. For example, if you feel leaden and weighted down when you're bored, a healthy counterbalance could be accessing levity by spending five minutes soaring on a child's swing set or floating in a pool. An unhealthy counterbalance would be seeking levity with substance use that disconnects you from your body.

Fear

I am afraid of . . . (you fill in the blank). She scares me. I feel flooded by fear.

It's no secret that all human beings know the particular resonance of fear: increased heart rate, sweaty palms, shallow breaths, laser focus, hypervigilance. The list goes on and on. Fear triggers the nervous system to the depth of its primal reptilian capacities. Mother Nature made sure that all creatures on earth were wired with the drive for survival, which includes a sensitive awareness toward anything that could potentially cause harm or bring danger to ourselves or our loved ones. Fear is essential on a primal level for humans and all other creatures. And, let's be honest, it can be a real buzzkill when you're aiming to feel carefree and happy.

Before we dig into the function of fear in relationships, let's get something straight: Fear is not the same as worry or anxiety. There can certainly be multidirectional overlap, but they are different. Here are my simplest definitions and distinctions:

- *Fear*: A primal response, encoded into the nervous system, that focuses entirely on keeping you alive, safe, whole, and out of danger's way. Fear is a process that exists in the present moment in response to something that is happening in the now. Fear is neurochemical and biological. It is solution-focused, meaning it looks for the quickest way to halt danger and regain safety.

- *Worry*: A psycho-emotional response to a potentially negative occurrence or experience most likely in the future. It is not necessarily based on facts or rationality, and it can be exacerbated by worst-case scenario thinking that is influenced by past experiences or traumas. There may not be an applicable solution for worry, and you may feel out of control, helpless, or hypervigilant as you await a negative outcome that may or may not ever arrive.

- *Anxiety*: A pathological form of worrying that includes rumination (repetitive thinking), hyperfocus (narrow awareness on negative possibilities), and physical sensations related to prolonged nervous

energy flowing through the mind and body (such as
a stomachache, a racing heart, insomnia, or an
uncomfortable buzzing sensation). Anxiety can be a
highly irrational, subjective, and distorted perception of something that others might not agree is a
big deal. It can be related to past trauma, personal
insecurity, or prolonged lack of perceived safety.

Now that those definitions are out of the way, let's talk more
about *fear*. Fear can show up in a person's relationships for many
different reasons. Here are a few common ones:

- Fear of losing someone they love by divorce, death,
  disloyalty, or rejection. This can easily catapult into
  worry and anxiety if the fear is prolonged, irrational
  or unfounded.
- Fear of emotional, physical, psychological, mental, or
  spiritual danger in an abusive or unhealthy
  relationship.
- Fear of confrontation, conflict, or hard conversations.
  Outside of the present-moment experience of fear
  when confrontation presents, this can also be an
  anxiety response where a person avoids such discomfort due to past negative experiences or worry
  about undesirable outcomes.
- Fear of vulnerability and potential rejection in moments of emotional intimacy and openness. This can
  also become an anxiety response if it is irrational,
  prolonged, or repetitive.

Fear is always a sign that something feels unsafe and danger
seems near. It is your nervous system's job to scan for potential
threats, but it is the job of your conscious mind to discern

whether your fear is rational, irrational, necessary to attend to, or irrelevant. The tricky part about the sensation of fear in relationships is that it can create a mind-body divide when your body senses danger that your mind believes is safe.

Carla's situation is a good example of such an inner conflict. A therapist herself, Carla spent years in personal counseling where she worked to extricate herself from a dysfunctional intimate relationship with Demmy that was filled with covert narcissistic abuse toward Carla. As she moved through layers of healing and awareness, finally able to end her long-term toxic relationship, Carla felt a strong desire to share all she had learned with her clients and community through social media and writing. Psychologically, it made sense for Carla to teach others the valuable skills she had acquired in her personal experience, combined with her clinical therapeutic skillset and training. She felt empowered and purposeful in aiding others who endured toxic relationships to break free and find healing. Her intention was to share valuable offerings with honesty and integrity without slandering Demmy in the least. Mentally, Carla felt capable, skillful, and strong in her capacity as a healer. Her body, however, felt differently.

When Carla considered the possibility that Demmy might see or read her teachings about toxic relationships and take them personally or feel in some way outed, her body reverted to a strong fear response. Throughout their relationship, Demmy had demanded that Carla remain silent about the abuse she underwent, and often he denied the existence of the abuse at all. It was only natural, therefore, for Carla to assume that Demmy would become incensed by feelings of humiliation at the knowledge that Carla was being vocal about topics that had remained covert between them for so long. After acknowledging the possibility that Demmy's aggressive tendencies could be triggered by her teachings, Carla spiraled deeper into fear. She worried that Demmy might pursue legal action toward her, however unfounded, for defamation of character or other such accusations that were never Carla's intention. Carla felt nauseous and shaky and even experienced insomnia and panic when she was caught in her body's layers of fear that so drastically opposed her mind's confidence.

What's a person to do when they are pulled in two such contradictory directions? Here's what Carla did: She developed a grounded plan from the perspective of her true Self somewhere in between the realistic fear that Demmy might act harmfully toward her and her spiraling worry that left her feeling powerless and fragile. From a perspective of true Self, Carla could discern that the risk of harm from Demmy was a small (though possible) scenario, so she thoughtfully assembled the protection of a legal team who would remain on deck just in case she needed them. With protective forces at her back, Carla courageously continued to teach the valuable offerings that felt aligned for her to share with her community. She provided countless people with support and resources to break free from their toxic relationships while soothing her own fear of attack from Demmy with proactive safety measures that would be ready for her if necessary.

The uncomfortable truth about fear in relationships is that yes, unfortunately, sometimes people do scary and harmful things to one another. Sometimes there is a very real threat that must be attended to. The good news is that as an adult, you have access to resources and all flavors of help and education that can support you once you discern the level of aid your fear response requires for safety. The key to accessing support for your nervous system is anchoring into true Self, where you can think rationally and reflect honestly. From there, you can strongly meet the needs of your inner system with supportive resources and nourishment.

When you venture inward and navigate relationally from the stable base of true Self, you may find that your fears are unwarranted and overdramatic. That's no problem! You can always release a deep exhale and dismiss fear from your mind and body when you realize that what you fear is not a true threat. But in the case where you discover the validity of your fear, true Self will always guide you toward the next right choice for self-support and safety.

> **How-To Tip** Draw a Fear monster. Consider including different metaphorical elements as you personify Fear. Is Fear large or small, human or alien? It may have a mouth full of teeth or perhaps be slithery like a snake that sneaks up on you. After drawing, journal about how Fear protects you by making itself scary. How does Fear keep you safe by diverting you away from threats? How does Fear wave a red flag in your face for your higher good? Notice rational and irrational ways Fear functions and how you respond.

Emotional Immaturity

You are so emotionally immature. I need an emotionally mature partner. You should be more emotionally mature by now.

Here is this week's lesson in not judging a book by its cover or a person by their external presentation: Someone who looks like a well-adjusted adult on the outside—appears to be high functioning, charming, and successful by all judgments of material wealth, status, and popularity—may or may not be truly mature in an emotional sense. Though they can manage a real estate empire, powerfully wield a physician's scalpel, or confidently speak to auditoriums full of people, emotionally immature people may completely lack the ability to access deep emotional connection and intimacy. They may also be unable to foster healthy conflict resolution when feelings get hurt and emotions ricochet sideways in relational dynamics. Not only can this be wildly triggering for a counterpart who is emotionally mature, but it can also be the tipping point between *mend* and *move on* that makes moving on seem like the healthiest option.

Dominic was a high-power attorney who frequently won and found himself on top of his industry in ways that affirmed his supremacy and influence. He dated freely without commitment or regard for his lovers, thoughtlessly spent big money at expensive locations, and looked to be a person who had figured out the nuance of successful adulting. One day Dominic showed up disheveled at my office, weary from a weekend of binging on substances and erotica in Las Vegas. On this day, he was finally able to observe his attachment to the materialism and inauthenticity he had been using to avoid the persistent emotional immaturity that lurked just beneath his surface presentation of Self. "How is it possible that I feel like a little boy in a power suit?"

Dominic and I worked together to identify and process the emotional immaturity that had tirelessly maintained his façade of adulthood. We discussed his avoidance of emotional intimacy, the way he used sexuality as a tool, and his flippant disregard for the feelings of both himself and others. Over time, Dominic learned to attended to his very young inner child who was steeped in shame and unhealed trauma. As he moved through the acknowledgment and ownership of his unhealed wounds that resulted in erratic and immature behavior, Dominic treaded the meaningful journey of stepping into true adulthood by cultivating a deep sense of maturity.

Dominic is a successful example. He noticed the chasm between his behaviors and his authentic Self and diligently worked to bridge the gap. Not everyone chooses to engage this work, as it requires profound courage and accountability to truly heal. Most people who are emotionally immature exist within the understanding that if they continually shunt accountability, live within the glass house of denial, and close their eyes to the maladaptive ways they engage in relationships, they will conveniently maintain a life where they can coast atop anything that might harm them. People like this treat others with reckless thoughtlessness, little to no empathy, and connection that is fueled by toxicity on many levels.

The sad reality of relating to a person who is deeply wounded yet unwilling to heal reflects the edges at which a relationship cannot be healthy without the genuine effort and participation of all involved. Often when a person finds themselves in a relationship with this kind of strife, they are in a dynamic with an *emotionally immature person (EIP)*. Dr. Lindsay C. Gibson is a clinical psychologist who literally wrote the book (well, actually books)[11] on the topic.

In her work, Dr. Gibson teaches that the development of maturity is not linear and can easily get derailed in certain facets while remaining intact in others. This is why emotionally immature adults are so often puzzling to figure out. They demonstrate harmful behaviors with certain people while presenting as wildly successful, popular, charming, and even famous in other arenas. This paradox demonstrates the difficult reality that it often takes a certain level of relational closeness and intimacy in order to get a true assessment of a person's level of emotional maturity. Being an adult, even an outrageously successful one, does not guarantee that a person has emotionally matured. Depending on their personal story and developmental trajectory, a person can seem adultlike in many functional capacities while remaining quite immature in the important relational territories of intimacy, empathy, and emotional connection.

If you are wondering how to tell if a person is an EIP or not, Dr. Gibson's research has identified five main characteristics of adult emotional immaturity:[12]

1. *Egocentrism*: This is when a person has difficulty seeing past themselves, their own perceptions, and their own feelings. They are the center of their universe to the detriment of acknowledging that other people are real and have feelings and perceptions that, though potentially different, may be valuable to consider.

2. *Limited empathy*: Empathy is the experience of feeling what you imagine another person feels in a given situation. It is based on emotional attunement and sensitivity that allows someone to place themselves in another's shoes and explore how it might feel to be them in an experience.

3. *Low capacity for self-reflection*: When I say *low* capacity, what I really mean is *low or no* capacity for self-reflection. Without the ability to turn curious awareness inward with the intention of knowing and understanding oneself, a person will not consider if they did something harmful, how they played a part in a dynamic, or what about themselves might require healing or growth. Without the capacity for self-reflection, a person is likely to project blame on anyone except themselves, embrace a victim mentality, and shunt all accountability.

4. *Emotional intimacy avoidance*: True connection between individuals is based on the mutual give-and-take of vulnerability, trust, care, and effort. If a person is unwilling to share about themselves, connect deeply with another, or give and receive emotional support, they vastly limit their potential for connection.

5. *Use of "affective realism"*: People who use affective realism design and rewrite reality to match what they feel it to be. They will deny the facts and feelings of other people in the service of supporting their own view of reality based on what they want to be true and how they see things.

If you read these words and note emotionally immature relationships in your own life or notice areas of emotional immaturity within yourself, try to simply receive this material as information. If you observe emotional immaturity within yourself, the good news is that you have full and complete control over your own growth trajectory. You can begin therapy, recruit a close friend or family member to talk with about your patterns, and delve into interior processing to healthfully rewire some of the relational patterns with those you feel close to. If you are now aware that an important person in your life exhibits emotional immaturity, it may not be so straightforward. Since most EIPs are unaware of their own emotional immaturity (ahem, affective realism), they likely will not be open to your defining them as such. The unconscious patterns and narratives that stunted their emotional maturity on the journey of their lives is something these individuals must heal in their own readiness—if they ever choose to. Please understand that it is not your responsibility to teach the emotionally immature adults in your life about their immaturity, nor is it your job to heal them. If they cannot healthfully relate to you by listening to your communications and noting your emotional experience, they may never be able to do so. You may need to distance yourself from a person like this for your own emotional health and safety (as well as your happiness and relational satisfaction) or even end the relationship.

In conclusion to this chapter, please remember that words are like spells: They can coax reality out of thin air simply by you uttering them, let alone by you believing in them. For better or worse, the words you choose to speak, hear, share, and internalize have deep impact on the construction of your internal identity and perspective of the world. If you are often triggered in one or many relationships, don't leap to the conclusion that they must all end. Your unhealed material likely contributes to why your trigger response is sensitive, and your counterpart's too. With mutual healing comes mutual soothing, and triggers cannot thrive in a relationship that is regulated and stable. The smoothest relation-ship sailing through triggering seascapes happens when both people are doing their own work, healing their own trauma and inner child wounds, and bringing their healthiest Selves into connection with one another. If you are working on your own healing and your counterpart refuses to do so, your unhealthy relationship will likely stumble on trigger after trigger as your nervous systems fail to gain emotional safety in the bond.

I am sure that along with the words shared in this chapter, you can think of others in your daily experience that may hold you back and limit you. Also consider your consistent usage of words that uplift and shape your life (and relationships) in positive ways. As with all things, you have immense choice about the words that impact and influence you. Are you choosing in alignment with your highest good?

How-To Tip In your journal, create two lists: one of words you frequently use or hear that negatively influence you and one of words that enliven and soothe you. Which list is longer? If too much negativity results from your language, you can change this by observing the pattern and choosing different words that positively impact you.

CHAPTER 7

Aligned Relationships

A Puzzle Piece Theory

Call to mind a puzzle: tens, hundreds, or even thousands of oddly knobbed and angled pieces that somehow fit together as a unified whole—but only after meeting proper alignment with one another. If you have ever patiently pieced together a puzzle, you're familiar with the deep satisfaction that comes when you find a piece that fits, likely after many attempts at aligning pieces that either blatantly oppose one another or almost (but not quite) fit. You also may be familiar with the irky feeling of trying to force the knobs of two misaligned pieces together. Since we don't tend to project much emotional material into puzzles, we don't typically feel the need to attach value judgments to the mismatched pieces, making them wrong or bad for not aligning. Disparity between pieces doesn't make one good and the other bad, or even your intentions to join them good or bad. It only indicates that they don't sync.

The same process of puzzling happens with relationships but with a whole lot more emotion and attachment involved. Because people are living, breathing, adaptive, growth-oriented, and dynamic beings (unlike puzzles), our fit and alignment with one another shift and change over time. This means you must release your attachment to *forever* in the context of relationships. Relational alignment reflects the congruence of two people's needs, values, capacities, and priorities in the present moment.

> **How-To Tip**   If you wonder how to recognize an aligned
> relationship, just ask your body. "Yes" or "no" thoughts might
> circle, but the malleable nature of the mind makes it unreliable
> when discerning true "yes" from true "no." Instead, turn to the
> body—a truth-teller by way of emotions and sensations. If you
> repeatedly notice tension, emptiness, or any other discomfort
> around a certain person, your body is indicating "no." Con-
> versely, a sense of ease, trust, or warmth indicates "yes." The
> more you listen to your body, the more familiar you will
> become with its nuanced communications.

If you have ever heard someone boast about a ten-, twenty-,
or fifty-year relationship (and maybe this has been you), such a
proclamation is typically spoken proudly. Are there long-term
relationships that demonstrate deep love, commitment, and
alignment? Absolutely. There are also long-term relationships
that have limped along unhealthily for years like a ragged ani-
mal in need of more than just a hearty meal. Such connections,
despite the marvel of their longevity, would have benefited from
ending long ago. Despite the warm, fuzzy feeling most of us experience when fantasizing about a lifelong ride-or-die relationship, a thirty-year dynamic filled with misery and resentment is
not something to aim for. Sometimes letting go and returning
to square one is the healthiest choice for all involved.

It is normal for relationships to move in and out of alignment
throughout time. That's not a problem. Instead, issues arise
when your attachment to the longevity of a relationship super-
sedes the quality of its alignment over time. You must be willing
to continually take stock of how a relationship feels and functions for all involved in order to truly ascertain its congruence.
In my experience, there are five main components of aligned
relationships, which I have organized into the acronym TRUST:

    1) T: True respect

People in a relationship must have mutual respect for each other's similarities, differences, uniqueness, and oddities. Without respect there is no foundation to build the connection upon.

2) R: Reciprocity

Every dynamic has a natural give-and-take flow between individuals. Although the flow can't always be exactly fifty-fifty, sharing and receiving must be balanced for a relationship to be sustainable.

3) U: Unwavering care

Relationships turn into cold, unloving entities without the proper amount of thoughtful care. Similarly to how most flowers need ample sunlight, human relationships require emotional warmth in order to thrive. When we see the messy parts of our loved ones and lean in anyway, unwavering care builds strength within the dynamic that fosters support and endurance—especially during challenging times.

4) S: Safety (physical, emotional, psychological)

Safety is a basic need for each and every person, regardless of how strong they may seem on the surface. We must feel that our bodies, minds, and hearts are protected and secure in order to be vulnerable in our most meaningful relationships if we are to truly benefit from connection. When any part of our system feels on guard and at risk, our heart remains protected and cannot flow freely.

5) T: Tandem values

Values are an important part of aligned relationships, even if they don't mesh completely. Differing opinions and beliefs can easily coexist as long as the relationship is congruent when it comes to values. For example, if one person values frequent in-person connection while the other needs more alone time and space, the value related to contact is misaligned and will likely cause problems. Differing opinions about how to spend money or which social circles to participate in may be less problematic because they do not always relate directly to the dynamic.

When puzzle pieces come together smoothly and a relationship feels aligned, it is akin to striking a resonant chord on a musical instrument that just feels right. Few experiences are as satisfying as the security and comfort of a truly aligned relationship. If you can call to mind one or two relationships of this type, you are fortunate indeed. Be sure to express your gratitude and appreciation for your aligned relationships regularly so your loved ones know how much they mean to you.

In the event of a misaligned relationship, sometimes a genuine conversation can bring it back online. We can unknowingly float astray from one another, caught up in the tides of life and distracted from our core connections. If both people are willing to listen, consider the other's perspective, and pivot toward better alignment, relationships can be repaired and grow to unimaginable heights and depths.

> **How-To Tip**   Never underestimate the power of the statement "Help me understand . . ." If you feel confused or uncertain about someone's needs, ask them to help you understand what they are. This is a potent tool for relational repair.

Sometimes letting go of a misaligned relationship is the healthiest action. Depending on your degree of comfort with confrontation, such a release can look like a passive floating away, a direct conversation, or something else entirely. Regardless of how you move away from an ill-fitting dynamic, please know that in the case of an irreparably misaligned relationship, letting go can free you both. If the relationship feels problematic for you, it is likely unhealthy for the other person as well, even if they cannot identify or acknowledge how. Despite three full tires, if a car has one flat tire the entire vehicle is endangered.

Letting go comes with a host of triggers and challenges unique to each individual's personal wounds. Sometimes guilt is associated with ending a relationship; other times a person may feel grief, fear, anger, relief, or any combination of emotions. They may remember past painful endings and associate the turmoil of such experiences with the present finale, or there may be a profound sense of freedom that an imbalance has been rectified. A question that can be helpful in allowing timely release is *Can someone else love each of us better?* It is powerful to remember that a major component of what brings us into relationship with one another is our desire for love, be it romantic or otherwise. When we let go of toxic, damaging, or problematic dynamics, we allow space for both parties to find healthier versions of what they need to feel meaningfully connected.

Walls

Right up front, I'll explain what I mean by *walls*. These are boundaries to the utmost degree—physical, emotional, and/or energetic barriers that keep people out. Walls are not there to be torn down. They exist for a very good reason and may even have saved your life at some point. A person's system constructs walls when they need extreme self-protection, so there is always a reason for their presence. If someone approaches the walls with curiosity and respect, they might have an opportunity to learn about why the walls exist. Treatment like this opens potential for repair in relationships. It is when a person approaches walls with a wrecking ball, viewing them as something to be forcibly removed, they only hunker down more strongly, remain unmoving, and grow in size and strength in response to the persistent threat.

It is true that people can sometimes prematurely erect walls in relationships that instead might benefit from more flexible boundaries, but that's not the topic of this section. This section explains the barriers we put in place between ourselves and others who cause harm or discomfort in our lives to such a degree that we feel the need to place them at a far distance from ourselves for protection and safety. Like the Great Wall of China, walls are not built in a day—or even a year or decade. Well, small walls can be, but the labyrinthine walls a person constructs for deep protection are most often constructed in response to lengthy relational cycling that causes trauma and deep harm. When you imagine a system of protective walls like a labyrinth, with your valuable Self at the cozy center, you get a visual picture of the multiple barriers a person can put in place to move another person, layer by layer, progressively further away from what matters most to them (their precious and vulnerable Self) until they finally reach the outside of the very last wall. At such a time, the offender stands beyond a barricade so final it may as well be the wall surrounding Troy (without a faulty opening for traitorous wooden horses).

Most people in my life would likely report, to varying degrees depending on their intimacy with me, that I am a warm person. I consider myself that way as well. Kindness is a dominant value of mine, along with generosity, compassion, and connection, among many others. That's what the world of Kate King feels like when a person is within the walls of my relational safety. The closer someone is to my true Self within the labyrinth of my protective structures, the more warmth and love they feel.

You may wonder why I build walls, and it's an excellent question. The answer is this: We all do. As human beings travel through life, we inevitably encounter people and experiences that feel unsafe, harmful, off-putting, or just icky. It's the natural way of relationships. They're not all good—not by a long shot. When your inner system perceives any kind of threat (real, imagined, or otherwise), it says to itself, *That was uncomfortable. I'll now do whatever I possibly can to avoid ever feeling this way again*. With the commitment to avoid repeating experiences that cause harm, walls are built as emotional, energetic, or physical measures toward separation. When painful experiences of the same (or similar) kind repeat despite the walls' existence, the walls grow higher and stronger. This can progress until the walls reach a magnitude where nothing that even has the smell of the harmful experience (or person) is permitted anywhere nearby. This is how we stay safe as living beings. Though not ideal, and certainly not the intention we bring into the beginning of new relationships, walls are essential in many cases. They can be both sanity-saving and, in extreme cases, lifesaving.

I once had a close primary relationship that created long-standing damage to my core Self in the form of deep psycho-emotional manipulation. This was an integral primary relationship with its origins stemming from long before I had developed even the beginnings of a labyrinth. Throughout decades of mal-treatment and violence, I placed an increasing number of walls between myself and this person. The attacks never ceased, and eventually my toxic counterpart landed outside the final wall of my fortress. From that vantage point she pummeled the wall with verbal abuse, gaslit like her life depended on it, defaced my character, and threw venomous slashes across my life choices and identity. She tried with all her might to bring my walls down with force, shame, and masterful manipulation. Nothing worked because the barricade had been strengthened and reinforced for so long. I had constructed something akin to a sophisticated artificial intelligence scanner that instantly closed all guards against this person. As this abuser kicked and screamed outside my walls, I remained calm and safe as I witnessed what had become of our relationship. I no longer collapsed under her pressure, no longer got hooked by her mind games, and no longer saw any hope for the future of our connection. This is when she accused me of being hard, harsh, and cold. "A goddess chiseled from stone" were her exact words at the time.

I considered what she said and reminded myself that the truth from her vantage point outside of my walls was true for her—even if I didn't agree. She wasn't making it up; she truly experienced me as a goddess chiseled from stone (whatever that really means). Then it occurred to me that it must actually feel cold and harsh outside of my walls. I've never been there myself, but I would guess that it feels similar to the cold desert of Siberia. Being removed from the warmth and generosity of my core must have been infuriating. It wasn't that I became hard and chiseled from stone, but that my walls formed such an effective protective system that they highlighted the stark distance between this aggressor and my authentic core Self. It's incredibly sad. I mourn for the loss that delivered the results of this experience, and yet I appreciate my walls.

When a relationship requires labyrinthine walls for protection and you still do not walk away from it, it indicates that the abuser has served as a core connection in your life. Truthfully, some relationships are easier to let go of than others. The degree to which you feel compelled to wall yourself off from another is important information when navigating any relationship, and especially when discerning how to release those that are deeply misaligned.

> **How-To Tip**   Grab any art materials you're comfortable with and draw your labyrinth of walls. Include yourself at the center and symbolically represent the person you wish to block. Then journal about your creative experience and note any emotional responses.

Dunbar's Number

From walls to circles, the following findings are from the work of British anthropologist Robin Dunbar, who scientifically proved that there is a number that captures the amount of meaningful connections a person can have in their life. This body of research is known as "Dunbar's Number,"[1] and it maps out as a series of concentric circles that represent various levels of relational intimacy. In their entirety, the circles allow space for about 150 stable relationships of varying emotional closeness and connection in a person's life. Consider your holiday card list or the guest list for a wedding or bar mitzvah. For many people, this number naturally hovers around 150. Consider the range of closeness you feel with every person in your life—from your most trusting and intimate confidante to the acquaintance you occasionally bump into but know little about. Each of our relational systems of concentric circles allows space for this range of intimacy for partners, family members, friends, coworkers, community members, neighbors, and acquaintances.

Visualize a map of four concentric circles that get progressively larger with each layer, looking like a dartboard. Specifically, Dunbar discovered that each layer can contain three times the amount of people as the prior layer: 5, 15, 50, 150. Additionally, each layer includes the people contained in the circles before it. This means that the fifteen tier-two connections include the five from your tier-one circle as well as ten more pretty good (but not tier-one-level) relationships. Due to the size of each ring, there are limitations for who and how many individuals can fit inside. Dunbar explains that in the innermost circle, what I call the "core circle," there is room for only three to five people. These are your ride-or-die besties, beloved family, and most trusted and intimate connections for whom you would walk through fire—and they would do the same for you. For me, my husband and two children take up three spots in my core circle, leaving two spots for dear friends. Not everyone will feel this way about their immediate family, leaving more spaces available for nonfamily connections.

With each progressive circle beyond the core, the level of emotional intimacy, trust, and dependency decreases, but space increases. This is why we can have far more acquaintances in our lives than best friends. It is also important to mention that people can jump circles. Someone who was once a fourth-tier acquaintance can become a third-, second-, or even first-tier connection if you mutually commit to enhancing the intimacy and priority of the relationship to build a meaningful bond. Oppositely, someone from your core circle can slide into second-, third-, or fourth-tier acquaintanceship if the connection weakens and no longer maintains the trust and reliability it once did. For this reason, it is important to be both intentional and flexible within the container of your relationships. Try to remain open to the possibility that a meaningful relationship from your past may have grown to be less crucial over time. Be clear about the present quality of each bond to consciously place connections in the circles where they truly belong. To simplify, here's how I think of the four circles:

- *Core circle, or tier one*: Ride-or-die, best of the best friends and closest family members. People with whom you feel deep, reliable trust and intimacy.
- *Tier two*: People you feel close to and perhaps see often and feel highly compatible with, but wouldn't call if something came up in the middle of the night.
- *Tier three*: People you might invite to a birthday party or weekend barbecue. You enjoy and feel connected to them, but you likely do not have depth or trust with them.
- *Tier four:* This is your weddings and funerals group who might attend your once-in-a-lifetime event, but probably not your sickbed with chicken soup.

In my personal work with mapping circles, I have found it necessary to reserve a specific corner outside of my dart board where I include an additional circle I call "deep space." This is where people who are a full-body *no* belong. Those who have abused and harmed me exist in this area of deep space, as do people who are invested in my smallness and wish negativity toward me. Deep space is a peaceful place where I assign no harm to these individuals, yet I consciously acknowledge that they lack the privilege of being relationally close to me.

How-To Tip   On your computer or by hand, create a map of four concentric circles. It should look like a dartboard. If you choose to include "deep space," add another circle near a corner of your page. Write every name of your 150 relationships within the circles, placing each person where they belong. If you need to, consult your contacts list. Visually represent where your relationships fall within the four (or five) circles so you can discern who is of greatest value and priority and whom you can give less effort and energy to. If you discover that you have been offering first-tier love to a fourth-tier relationship, that signals you to get honest with yourself about whether that relationship is worth the energy you feed it. Conversely, if you have been treating a first-tier person with third- or fourth-tier effort, you might consider stepping up your game to preserve the value of that relationship. Remember to use a pencil for this exercise. You'll be glad for the ability to erase if people jump circles in the future.

Bargaining

Glennon Doyle, author and influencer, speaks[2] about particularly alarming advice she received from her marriage therapist as she worked through relationship issues with her ex-husband. In response to Doyle's confession that she could not bring herself to have sex with her husband, the therapist recommended that she should consider giving him oral sex instead. To this astounding recommendation, the therapist added that this suggestion works well for many women, as it can be considered less intimate. Hold the phone, drop the mic, do whatever you need to do to pull your jaw up off the floor and reign in your disbelief that anyone, let alone a therapist, would offer advice like this with a straight face. Lesson number one: Don't trust opinions from just anyone, even if they are a licensed professional in a position of power. Lesson number two: Downgrading your degree of self-abandonment from one unhealthy level to another is still self-abandonment with no exceptions.

When your mind, body, heart, and whole being tell you through any form of inner communication (viscerally, emotionally, cognitively, or with any other sensation) that a relationship feels wrong, icky, harmful, or misaligned for you, the answer is not to find a more tolerable way to stick with the status quo. Asking yourself to soldier on in a dynamic that is not good for you is not the answer. Not now, not ever.

If your compliance within a relationship (be it maritally, with family, professionally, or socially) has caused you harm or discomfort, you have likely played into the dynamic with your best efforts to keep the peace and avoid upsetting someone or losing something you care about. People-pleasing and relational inauthenticity do not deliver long-term sustainable results for healthy, lasting dynamics. When you engage from a place of fear or hypervigilance, tolerating maltreatment or unhappiness for the sake of peacekeeping, you participate in constructing a dynamic that hurts you instead of heals you. Bargaining with yourself to trade one unhealthy behavior for another in order to maintain the dysfunction with a grain more comfort is not the solution. Situations like these require dramatic (sometimes radical) change such as confrontation, truth-telling, new boundaries, or endings.

My client Jose chose to go no-contact with his father after years of verbal and physical abuse that he worked tirelessly to heal through years of therapy and self-reflection. When he was finally ready to pull away from his father, Jose was met with strong coercion from his mother, who blamed Jose for her stress-induced physical symptoms, like heart palpitations and insomnia, that stemmed from her internal reaction to his decision. She accused Jose of causing harm to her and could not understand that his choice was being made for self-protection. In a fit of bargaining, Jose's mother begged him to resume contact with his abusive father and return to collapsing within the perpetually harmful dynamics of their relationship so that she could feel better and sleep soundly once again. As Jose proceeded with his estrangement from his father, his mother lashed out further with guilt, shame, and malicious comments that demonized Jose as the sole problem of the family system. She tried every maneuver imaginable to return Jose to his prior role in the family that maintained the homeostasis they had come to know as normal.

Jose disrupted the comfortable (though unhealthy) family norm when he said "no more" and chose to walk away from the insidious abuse he had tolerated all his life. Rather than interpreting his decision as a protective response to the harm they had caused, Jose's family was unable to self-reflect and approach the situation with the curiosity necessary for repair. Thanks to the layers of deep inner work Jose had done, he saw their lashing out, blame, and bargaining for what they were: desperate attempts to return the unhealthy family system to its predictable rhythm. When Jose acted to protect himself, his decision thrust his parents into the uncomfortable experience of facing problems they never intended to face and still lacked any desire to heal. Their preference to blindfold themselves to the truth Jose reflected with his actions demonstrated their unwillingness to do the necessary work to foster genuine love toward their son with the humility and effort that was required for them to admit that their dynamic was, in fact, corrupt.

Jose never got the relational mending he hoped for in his family of origin. His parents persistently resisted participation in reparative work with him. Jose ended up losing his father by choice, his mother by her unwillingness to honestly see the situation, and several colluding siblings and extended family members who were unable to extricate themselves from the conditional safety of a distorted family. Additional people who witnessed the collapse between Jose and his biological family from the sidelines consciously or unconsciously remained compliant with the family's unhealthy patterns with their lack of action. Some even used bargaining by trying to convince Jose that staying in a harmful situation and taking the path of least resistance was favorable for the family at large, arguing that tolerating abuse benefited the family by keeping drama at bay. This *You're okay, it's not that bad* response was manipulative gaslighting that Jose was finally ready to gracefully sidestep after years of being convinced to question himself by the people he trusted most. On some level, these individuals, too, found it more comfortable to tiptoe around in denial and avoidance than run the risk of drawing negativity toward themselves by admitting that the issues were real, wrong, and harmful.

Deposits and Withdrawals

Humans are a lot like banks. There is a constant influx and outflow of energy, resources, effort, time, and care embedded in the habits of each person. When it comes to the flow of in and out between people, it's like two banks each supporting each other's cash flow balance. If one person makes withdrawals from the other to the exclusion of making equivalent deposits, they soak up the majority of the relationship's resources like time, effort, and care. The imbalance of a dynamic like this makes the interplay unsustainable for the person on the giving end. This is where reciprocity comes in.

It is certainly unrealistic to have a precise fifty-fifty dynamic of giving and taking between two people all the time, like when I shared Cheerios with my dog as a child: *one for you, one for me.* Realistically, it looks more nuanced in adult relationships: *one for you, three for me. Four for you, one for me.* The important thing is not that every give-and-take is noted in the ledger with rigid fairness, but that over time the reciprocity is more or less equal. When both people get their needs met, it implies that mutual respect and attention are being paid to the balance of reciprocity.

It is with this kind of general fairness that the connection be-tween people can most positively and healthfully contribute to someone's life.

For almost twenty years, my best friend and I have met every week for a walk-and-talk. Luckily for us we are both therapists, so our walks can sometimes feel therapeutic. On other more lighthearted days, it's the banter of two women who deeply cherish one another. In the time we carve out for weekly con-nection, my friend and I both feel safe to share our struggles, concerns, issues, joys, milestones, and confusions. Our walks are not structured rigidly with *ten minutes for you, ten minutes for me*. Sometimes one of us requires several consecutive walks to take up the majority of the space. This works for two reasons:

- First, we are both strongly aware of the space we use. If we notice that we need more time to share and process, we acknowledge the need and ask the other person if it feels okay for them. Sometimes we may even ask each other, *Do you have space to support me with this?* And the answer "no" is always allowed.
- Second, we both prioritize reciprocity. Even when one of us needs to take more space, we always re-member that although our conversations may feel like therapy at times, they are not therapy. In therapy, the client has a one-way relationship with the thera-pist, and reciprocity is not required (or appropriate). Therapy is a paid transaction for psycho-emotional and mental health support. Friendship is not therapy. It requires reciprocity, even if both parties are therapists.

Reciprocity is necessary in friendship, partnership, family re-lationships, work relationships, and all other kinds of relationships that are not based on appropriate paid transactions. This does not necessarily mean that you will find it easy to engage all of your connections with reciprocity without working at it— sometimes it takes intention and effort to cultivate a balanced dynamic. Certain people habitually lean more toward being the *givers* in a relationship while others tend toward being *receivers*. People who are used to caring for others or acting from unhealed fawning or people-pleasing tendencies can easily fall into the trap of nonreciprocity by overgiving. Those more predisposed to emotional immaturity or with narcissistic tendencies may become overly comfortable with receiving. These dynamics can be modified and updated when both participants acknowledge the pattern and work toward changing it.

Not all relationship participants, however, want to change an imbalanced dynamic. It can be highly seductive for a person who gains multitudes of what they need without having to work very hard to give much back. Why would they? Such a shift would require their willingness to compromise by receiving less and expending more effort to give more, which may not come naturally to them. Whether a person is consciously resistant to such a pivot or not, whether they feel capable of compromise of this kind or not, imbalanced relationships rarely last long.

Before my client Remy had done much of his relational healing, he had a friendship in early adulthood where he frequently showed up as a people-pleaser who rarely said "no." Despite Remy's positive intentions, he was confused about the difference between people-pleasing and kindness, thinking they were the same. They are not. Kindness is based on honesty and integrity. It reserves the right to say "no" and set respectful boundaries. People-pleasing is a behavior born from the "fawn" nervous system response, which assumes that saying "yes" and keeping others happy is the only ticket to safety. People who default to

people-pleasing probably had to work hard at earning and se-
curing love in childhood. These individuals likely developed a
core belief that love is highly conditional and must be won by
exhibiting certain *good* or *right* behaviors. Remy's confusion led
him to cultivate several relationships that held dishonesty in
their foundations. Remy's friends had no idea that the way he
was showing up, seemingly willing and generous, was dishonest; how could they? That was Remy's responsibility, not theirs.
Over time he set the unsustainable expectation that he would
say "yes" to most things, and if he said "no" it meant they should
keep asking until he caved in and reverted to "yes."

I can relate to Remy's experiences, particularly with a friendship from years ago where my friend became very sick and suddenly required immense effort and care from her closest connections. Since I had unintentionally been dishonest about my
availability and boundaries all along, she believed I could be
counted on as a core person to help her navigate her challenging circumstances. This lasted only until it combusted, if you
know what I mean. I could not sustain this friend's expectations.
At the time, direct conversations terrified me, so the best I could
do was to talk about our relationship through the metaphor of
houseplants. It went a little something like this:

> *Me*: If we were houseplants, I would be a succulent and you
> would be a leafy green pothos.
> *Friend*: Okaaay . . .
> *Me*: I think you need to be watered more often than I can water
> you. And I need much less watering than this relationship
> provides. [I was cryptically expressing that I needed less con-
> tact than my friend needed.]
> *Friend*: Okay. How much watering do you need?
> *Me*: I need to be watered only like once every few months, and
> you seem to need watering weekly. I can't keep up.

Friend: But this is a friendship, and it's our job to keep each other watered.

Me: Yes, but we each need different amounts of water. 1 am drowning here, and 1 can't sustain how thirsty you are.

Friend: Sometimes in friendship you have to water the other one more than you want to.

Me: 1 can't.

Friend: 1 don't understand. You have always watered me as much as 1 needed.

Me: 1 know. 1 am sorry. 1 didn't know how to tell you 1 couldn't keep up with that.

My metaphor basically worked to explain the conundrum at hand, but the relationship didn't survive. We were unable to find a pivot that worked for us both, and our bond ended. It is my hope that by terminating a dynamic where neither of us was getting our true needs met, we both became free to find others who could more honestly meet our connection needs. 1 hope with all my heart that this was the experience for my old friend. Sometimes relational problems like these result from unhealed inner wounds in one or both participants. Other times it may simply be a misalignment of personality, lifestyle preferences, or introversion/extroversion.

1 have learned to feel proud of my introvert tendencies, despite the opinion of many an extrovert that introversion is a form of pathology (it's not, by the way; it is a temperament that the Myers-Briggs Company has found in 56.8% of the population).[3] January 2nd has even been named World Introvert Day to honor the many people in society who would much rather fly under the radar than have any type of day dedicated to them. One book that helped me own and appreciate my introversion is *Quiet: The Power of Introverts in a World That Can't Stop Talking*[4] by Susan Cain. With the combination of her work and other

resources, I have learned to see my social selectiveness, inner-reflective tendencies, sensitivity, and relational attunement as strengths, even as they differ from the gifts of an extrovert. That being said, I have had experiences (in addition to the one with the pothos friend) where my introversion clashed loudly with the extroverted needs of another. In some scenarios we were able to find a healthy compromise to maintain connection, and in others the relationships found their natural endings.

> **How-To Tip**   Where are you on the introvert/extrovert spectrum? And yes, it is a spectrum. You don't have to pick a side, and one is not better or worse than the other. Introverts don't hate people—they simply recharge in solitude while extroverts recharge in the company of others. On a scale from one to ten, with one being "extreme introvert" and ten being "extreme extrovert," plot yourself.

Relational compatibility is a complex, multifaceted science experiment that takes time, awareness, and intention. Be gentle with yourself as you bumble along. Try new things and potentially find yourself in uncharted territory within your relationships. As you grow and develop through your lifespan, you will change. New layers of healing and awareness will provide different possibilities for your connections with others and with your Self. Simply notice and be present with the You you are in the present moment without attaching to past Selves or future ideals. If a relationship syncs and feels good to your heart, mind, and body, by all means continue along that path. When something feels misaligned, icky, or uncomfortable to the Self you currently are, it is your responsibility as the CEO of your system to make alterations accordingly.

CHAPTER 8

Parts Psychology

How Your Parts Feel About Their Parts

This book is squarely centered around your relationships with others, so let's direct the conversation toward how *parts psychology* accounts for the smattering of possible effects that can ignite when different ancestral lineages join together (and possibly make babies together) in relationships that involve your heart, mind, body, and soul.

If you have been maneuvering around your relationships under the assumption that there is only one single You interacting with your loved ones, you have been mistaken. In fact, you are a crucial yet individual link in the very long chain of your family line. Not only are you the singular link that interacts with others in your own chain, but you also mingle with links in the chains of lineages outside of yours when you build relationships with other people who are not your family. Various recent psychological methodologies (Internal Family Systems being my personal favorite) have discovered that each person is comprised of one true Self and many parts. If you think about it, I'll bet you can remember a time when you sensed your internal system, saying something like, *Part of me feels really bad about my colleague's face-plant on the sidewalk, but part of me thinks maybe it's karma because they're constantly rude to everyone at the office.* And you would be correct, because your thinking successfully identified two conflicting parts of yourself (neither of which are your true Self, by the way) that disagree about the justice and vindi-cation of another person's situation.

You may be wondering where parts come from and why they are not true Self. As we surf the waves of life, elements of our inner system fractal off into adaptive parts that respond to the challenges life presents at different stages. This fragmentation process is both natural and universal, so there's no need to pathologize it. Having many parts is quite different from hav-ing multiple personalities or other forms of acute mental illness and psychosis. Every person's inner relationship between parts and Self is a delicate dynamic of protection and adaptation as we work to remain safe and whole in an ever-changing (and some-times threatening) world. Parts can look like common arche-types from the collective unconscious[1]—the Sage, the Wounded Child, the King/Queen, or the Villain. They can also be specific to your personal patterns, such as the Perfectionist, the Angry Part, or the People-Pleaser. Additionally, you may relate to cer-tain characters in movies or stories that you feel represent cer-tain parts of you such as Gandalf the Grey (from Lord of the Rings), Eeyore (from Winnie-the-Pooh), or the Evil Queen (from Sleeping Beauty).

Without delving too deeply into the psychology of parts work—if you'd like a deeper dive into this methodology, read my book *The Radiant Life Project*—it is important to know the fun-damental difference between your true Self and your many parts: *True Self* is the most basic essence of who you are with-out the weights and wounds of your fears, traumas, distortions, and other residue that evidence life's hardships. Internal Family Systems identifies eight qualities of Self: compassion, creativ-ity, curiosity, connectedness, courage, clarity, calmness, and confidence.[2] Sensing the 8 C's within yourself indicates that you are presently relating to yourself and others from a true Self perspective. Because dialing in to all 8 C's can feel overwhelming, I tend to default to compassion and curiosity as a litmus test to determine whether I am anchored in true Self or not. When I have floated astray into the realm of parts, those are my two qualities of Self that nosedive first. If I cannot access compassion or curiosity in response to whatever (or whomever) the moment holds, I know I'm not operating from true Self. From this vantage point I'll likely come to see that an adaptive part of me has taken the wheel to protect me from whatever threat it believes may come from my present experience.

Here's a real-life example from one of my clients: In a tense moment when Susannah is trying to get her kids ready for school, she might be flooded by Efficiency and Time-Stickler parts—especially if the kids are running a few minutes behind. Susannah might be snappy with her children about getting their backpacks packed and shoes tied, and her adrenaline might be pumping. In a moment like this, Susannah's parts would be flooding her system because they believe that being on time and not missing the school bus is the most important thing in the world. If her kids missed the bus, she would have to deal with the consequences of driving them to school, waiting in the torturous drop-off line, and likely being late for a meeting, which would set her day askew. If Susannah could mindfully observe her parts for what they are—efficient and time-oriented—she might see their function and protective nature. Susannah might choose to cultivate gratitude for her parts, compassion for their struggle, and curiosity about whether their fears are really that big of a deal. By observing them in such a way, Susannah will have found true Self and no longer be driven exclusively by her Efficiency and Time-Stickler parts. From true Self, Susannah could acknowledge the importance of timeliness while also remembering that missing the bus isn't the end of the world. She would likely choose to speak kindlier to her children, help them get out the door, and cool down her anxious nervous system to meet the day more calmly.

> **How-To Tip** What are your dominant two or three C's of Self? In your journal, explore the 8 C's (courage, compassion, clarity, curiosity, connectedness, courage, calmness, and confidence). Note how they show up in your life (and with whom), when you most often experience the different qualities, and which you feel are most easily accessible to you during times of stress.

The defining quality of *parts* is that they are adaptive. By *adaptive* I mean that your parts represent fragments of your internal system that evolved to match and counteract whatever threat(s) you were faced with at the age when the part was created. For example, I learned very early that getting in trouble was the absolute worst thing that could happen to me. It wasn't a child's normal *aw, shucks* response to getting in trouble but more like an *AH! The world is ending!* irrational response. Getting in trouble was something I deeply feared because I believed that it would threaten my safety and existence. Still to this day, there's a squirmy tension and heavy block that forms in my stomach when I step a toe out of line or upset someone. When I spy a police officer on the highway, I instinctively slam on my brakes—even if I am driving the speed limit. I am not in true Self in moments like these. My system is being flooded with the fearful energy of my Good Girl part that desperately wants me to avoid getting in trouble (or getting a speeding ticket) in order to remain safe. When the Good Girl part formed during my preschool days, my psyche constructed it because I needed an inner mechanism I could rely on to help me follow the rules, keep my controversial feelings to myself, and remain anticipatory of others' needs. As long as my Good Girl part was in charge, I would never feel the absolute terror that came with getting in trouble. I can now recognize the Good Girl, and (mostly) prevent her energy from flooding my system, but for a long time she served as a dominant shield for what I perceived to be life's greatest threats: punishment and rejection. Keep in mind, not all threats to your Self are obvious or even rational. You are equipped with a unique internal village that knows how to keep itself safe, secure, whole, and alive, and it will take any measure necessary to do so.

Parts work deeply impacts relationships when two people's inner systems, complete with all of their component parts along with their true Selves, link to form a meaningful emotional connection that places their parts and Selves in intimate connection with each other. That's where fireworks happen, for better or worse. If one person enters a relationship with a dominant part that craves attention while the other person enters with a part that requires solitude, the relationship will encounter a big issue if those two parts remain front and center.

In addition to the Good Girl part, another of my dominant parts that tends to take the stage during stressful moments is a rigid, micromanaging part I fondly call Type-A Acrobat. She's an extremely adaptive part of me that learned early on to make leaps and maneuvers (hence *acrobat*) to double down on getting stuff done with nearly superhuman efficiency. As an added dimension, my Type-A Acrobat can also catapult beyond me and project toward others who trigger my stress response. When my system is flooded by my Type-A Acrobat, I cannot feel compassion for the loved one I am relentlessly micromanaging (apologies to my husband), nor can I access curiosity about why that person might behave as they do. In this flooded state, true Self is buried beneath a pile of protective wards and charms

manufactured by my hypervigilant Type-A Acrobat who functions to control the situation in order to protect me. This inner
dynamic plays out because long ago, Type-A Acrobat developed
a narrative like *As long as I keep everything controlled and moving
smoothly, I'll be safe.*

Here's how all this language about parts and true Self relates
to you: Each and every one of your personal, professional, intimate, and casual relationships exist in a teeter-totter of parts-
to-Self balance, personally and interpersonally. We all constantly
field signals to determine if we are safe or in danger. If our system identifies a threat of any kind, it will bring the most
convenient or competent part forward to handle the presenting danger. This process unfolds while we simultaneously react to different iterations of similar experiences in our relationships. That's a lot to manage, and it is why relationships can
feel so complex—because they are.

As ideal as it would be for two people to both be firmly anchored in true Self while relating to one another, it is not possible all the time for anyone. True Self is not a final destination;
it is a home base from which you float astray and must learn to
return to. To connect IFS parts work with the polyvagal theory
of the nervous system, true Self lives in ventral vagal activation—
the state of being that is grounded, calm yet energized, and
centered in presence. The beautiful thing about each and every
one of your parts, as distorted and dysfunctional as they may
seem, is that they carry exquisite intelligence that allows them
to adapt to life's challenges. They also maintain the positive intention of taking care of you in the only way they know how
because they love you. This is why the goal is not to eradicate
any parts or label them *bad* or *wrong*, but to unburden them
from the protective measures they believe they must heroically
fulfill. Healing the original wound that resulted in the develop-

ment of a part allows the part itself to reintegrate healthfully in your system. Then it can lower its shield and weaponry and remove the pressure to single-handedly protect you. From an integrated perspective, a part can observe that you have grown into a strong, capable adult and realize that you are no longer the vulnerable child you once were who desperately needed its protection.

You see, parts become frozen in the time when they are created. They do not know when your growth and maturity no longer require their vigilance toward the specific threats they feel compelled to protect you from. A child who lives in a physically abusive household might develop a part that drives them to be agreeable and meek in order to remain safe from the abuse that ensues when they speak out or stand up for themselves. If this child grows into an adult who no longer lives with the threat of abuse, their protective part may continue to feel compelled to behave with the agreeableness and meekness from childhood as a safety measure, even when the threat no longer presents. In this case, healing requires that the person recognizes their foundational safety in adulthood. When this person teaches their system that they have become a strong, capable adult who can self-protect and consciously choose safe relationships, the defending part no longer needs to tirelessly guard them.

How-To Tip   When conflict arises and you get triggered and reactive (increased heart rate, elevated temperature, internal pressure, whatever your personal signals are), pause. Rather than reacting impulsively from the perspective of your adaptive part, breathe deeply three times and/or walk away from the conversation. Is the trigger actually in the room with you? Does the other person remind you of someone who is not currently present? When you feel calm, return to the conversation and share your awareness with the other person if it feels safe. It can be healing to calmly process the experience together and educate your loved ones about your adaptive parts so that they can better support you if/when the experience repeats.

Are You My Mother?

The 1960 children's book *Are You My Mother?*,[3] written by P. D. Eastman, a mentee of Dr. Seuss, tells the tale of a lost little bird. The story's protagonist is freshly hatched from its egg and has fallen from its nest, and it takes the reader on a heartfelt pursuit of finding its mother. The small creature approaches a hen, a kitten, and even what it calls a "snort" (i.e., a large tractor that makes loud snorting noises). It innocently asks each of them, "Are you my mother?" The animals (and the "snort") all respond that no, they are not the mother the lost bird seeks. As is common in children's books, all ends well for the tiny creature. Our heroic little bird eventually discovers that its mother simply dashed off to find the chick a bite to eat, so no harm no foul.

Even as the idealism of children's books appeals to the lost little ones within us (our inner child parts), most adults understand that real life doesn't always shake out with well-resolved happy endings. Sometimes the motherly love (or spousal love or caring friendship) our inner children needed was harshly betrayed, withheld, revoked, or never given in the first place, and the wounds run deep. Such profound relational pain can carry from childhood into adulthood, persisting until long after our baby teeth fall out and gray hair makes its unwelcome appearance upon our adult heads.

I remember a poignant therapy session I had during a pivotal time when I sought to fill the absence of a crucial relationship I had ended for my mental health and emotional safety. Though estrangement from this toxic person was undoubtedly healthy, the void their absence left behind was stark. It was an irreplicable relationship, despite my efforts to secure a place-holder bond I hoped could meet my existential longing for un-conditional love and support. My therapist and I mused at my relatability to the helpless little bird from the story, courageously approaching so many misaligned creatures with the hope of constructing Mother from personalities that simply couldn't fill the little bird's need.

Unluckily for me, I didn't return to the nest to find that the person I had been seeking was available to me. What I did dis-cover, however, was that I was wrong to identify myself as a helpless little bird when in reality I had grown into a majestic owl. You see, I had spearheaded my emotional search for belong-ing and safety with my Wounded Inner Child part rather than tending to that scared part with the security and strength of my adult true Self. Sure, that fragile little bird still exists within me and will always endure as a younger Me who experienced life through her perspective, but there's no reason why she should be in charge of my inner system—that's a job for true Self. My Wounded Inner Child harbored the unfortunate lesson she learned from her experience that love doesn't come for free—it must be earned with compliance and smallness. Until a trust-worthy adult (in the form of Self) circled back to unburden her from trying to stay protected by the wisdom of her lived expe-rience (as distorted it was), my Wounded Inner Child believed she had to fulfill a protector role by sparing me from the pain she felt.

The good news is that I no longer dominantly embody that young part of me. I have grown into my developed Self through years of reparative inner work and corrective experiences. In the past when I was flooded with the energy of my wounded part, I unconsciously embodied her fear, fragility, and desperation. It was not until I tucked her securely under the protective wing of my elder owl Self, my true Self, that I embraced the deep knowing that I have grown into the trustworthy, reliable support my inner child yearned for but never received until now.

Let's stick with the owl analogy a while longer. Did you know that owls cough up pellets to expel the indigestible material from their meals? As a child in nature camp, I hunted in the grass for the soft pebble-sized gray bundles and brought them to the lab for dissection. Upon opening a pellet of hardened fur and feathers, my friends and I excavated entire skeletons of tiny mice and other creatures that had been the owl's meal. The sophisticated digestive system of this remarkable bird was designed in such a way that after the essential nutrients were absorbed from a feeding, everything else would be discarded for the health of the bird's system. Wow, right?

If you're still with me, following this lengthy teaching, you may recognize that coughing up pellets of indigestible material is an essential aspect of what conscious Self work does in the service of unhealed parts. Self absorbs the vital nourishment we were fed (love we received, important lessons we learned, healthy beliefs we constructed, etc.) and rids our systems of anything we took in that we would be better off without (unhealthy narratives, toxic beliefs about ourselves and the world, damaging people or values). In this way, Self offers healthy release and clearing for younger parts that did not know how to do so for themselves. This, my friends, is the power of parts work in action.

How-To Tip   Applying the metaphor of owl pellets, how have you refused to digest certain material that was fed to you? Journal or create art about what this brings up. Draw a dissected gray owl pellet with images inside that represent your outdated relationships, belief systems, cultural narratives, or personal values. For 3D art, use yarn to depict the owl pellet, and weave small statues, collage words, and other tokens through the yarn to represent indigestibles from your past that you wish to release.

Parts Work in Adult Relationships

As discussed, parts get created as life happens—especially in the most challenging periods when we get destabilized and freaked out. As you note your different parts and acknowledge which have embodied dominant roles for protection and heroism, consider asking yourself three important questions:

1. *Who did you see do this?* Who in your life (likely in childhood) did you see exhibit the behaviors you have tailor-made into your own way of existing in the world? Think about parents and early caregivers, mentors and teachers, adults you admired, parents of close friends, or any others who had an early influence on you.

2. *Who did this to you?* You may have come into direct contact with someone who impactfully projected their unhealed wounds onto you, victimized you in large or small ways, or harmed you consciously or unconsciously.

3. *How did this behavior help you meet your needs?* Think back and consider the adaptive function of this behavior during a time when you may have felt small and powerless, insecure, or confused. How did this behavior help you fit in, survive, stay safe, fly under the radar, maintain control, or fulfill other functions deemed crucial by your younger You?

Example time: I am familiar with a part of myself that I call The Judge. As you might guess, The Judge is the part of me that thinks in black and white about wrong vs. right, good vs. bad, acceptable vs. unacceptable. This part can be righteous, shaming, and belittling when in its full glory. It judges both myself and others, and I have greatly increased my awareness of it in my inner work journey. Here is how the three questions apply to my version of The Judge:

1. *Who did you see do this?* I witnessed the collective of my biological family embody The Judge on a regular basis. I grew up in a family that used a great deal of nonverbal communication to nudge each member toward the family's definition of right/good and away from wrong/bad. My greater family system operated under many assumptions that insinuated who we had to be, how we were required behave, what we were supposed to and not supposed to say, and what we needed believe if we wanted to belong. There was little room for individuation and autonomy in a system that thrived on codependency and enmeshment fostered by control and power dynamics under the guise of "respect" and "rightness."

2. *Who did this to you?* As mentioned, my biological family was strict in their messaging about who I was supposed to be and how I was required to behave. I both witnessed my family members' versions of The Judge in action and was the recipient of their rulings. The singularity of "rightness" became unavoidably clear when I left home to attend college and made choices outside of the family groupthink that they disagreed with. When I asserted autonomy and tried

to be my true Self, the contrast with our family's rules was glaring. In an attempt to nudge me back in line, I was treated with great resistance and ongoing emotional violence in an attempt to realign me with the collective system's opinion of good/right related to my career, lifestyle, behavior, and relationship choices.

3. *How did this behavior help you meet your needs?* Being raised in a system that clearly delineated who, how, and what I had to be in order to earn love and belonging, I developed The Judge to hold that line for myself internally (and it got projected externally too). I learned that there was a clear "good," a clear "bad," and no nuanced gray zone in between. Although I ultimately bucked the system I came from by embodying true Self regardless of my family's harsh punishment, it took me a long time to appreciate The Judge. At first, I was unsure of how to honor The Judge's clarity and decisiveness while also kindly removing it from the driver's seat of my life. Now I consult with The Judge when I need help with discernment, but I no longer default to The Judge's perception and harsh ruling without conscious intention.

Here's the takeaway I want you to integrate from this section: We all have parts. They are adaptive, and they show up all over our relationships like the spots of a dalmatian. Sometimes this works well, when a healthy part of me feels connected to a healthy part of you, and together we thrive and bring out the best in each other. But what happens when a wounded part of Jane, for example, confronts, reacts to, and clashes with a wounded part of her brother Frank? Or when Jane's unhealed part cannot love and appreciate Frank's healed part because of the discomfort it instigates in her? Sticking with The Judge as an example, it could be problematic if both Jane and Frank have inner Judges who cannot agree on what is fair, just, and right within their sibling dynamic. Another problematic scenario would be if one party's Judge conflicts with a part in the other that prizes spontaneity and free spiritedness. Situations like these clearly demonstrate that many (if not all) relational conflicts are based on clashes between parts. The problem with relating to each other from the perspective of parts is that when we are flooded with the energy of a part's adaptations to its life circumstances, true Self is nowhere in sight. Remember, even though certain parts do a decent job of helping us maintain everyday functioning in this crazy game we call Life, it's only from true Self that we can connect and relate authentically while remaining compassionate and curious toward those who are different from ourselves.

If you can identify the parts of yourself and whomever else is at play in your undesirable dynamic, you will more easily heal the issue—at least your role in the issue—by intentionally returning to true Self. It is only when you recognize that you are being flooded by a part that you can regain the capacity to recognize that the part is not wholly who you are—it is simply the adaptive mechanism you are unconsciously bringing forward to meet the situation at hand. Once you observe your maladaptive part as a well-intentioned aspect of your psyche, simply doing what it knows how to do based on what life has taught it, you can step back from that perspective and offer your inflamed part the compassion and care it desperately needs from true Self. It's a lot like a parent witnessing their child's temper tantrum with love and understanding rather than getting caught up in the idea that the tantrum represents the entirety of their child.

When you practice noticing the parts at play within yourself and others, you gain valuable information about the unhealed wounds you have likely been carrying for a very long time. Acknowledging your inner work at this level makes it easier to love the messier parts of yourself as well as any others you may have long rejected and reacted toward. There is an important boundary implicit in this recognition, however. Although it is healthy to be aware of the wounds your loved one's inner children carry, it is not your job to heal them on their behalf—nor is such a thing possible. Each person's healing is their own responsibility and must be unlocked by the mature presence of their own capable adult Self. Intimate relationships can certainly bring someone's baggage into the light for awareness and processing, and you can absolutely hold patience and compassion in your heart toward the unhealed material of your loved ones, but do not think that because you feel close to someone you are in any way responsible for repairing their wounded parts.

Herein lies the tricky business of adult relationships. You must learn how to be vulnerable and honest with those you care about regarding the baggage you carry and inner work you still have yet to heal while not projecting that responsibility beyond yourself. Also, you must compassionately witness the unhealed material within your loved ones without leaping to fix or heal it for them. Yikes, I know. This is a huge relationship pitfall that tends to create mega strife between people. A common misunderstanding that ties relationships into knots is that people do not always understand the limits of *caring about someone*. Many people have developed parts like The Caregiver, The Lover, or The Over-Giver that contribute to the false belief that people are projects to be undertaken. Parts like these mistakenly believe that when you commit to another person you also commit to healing them. Realistically, the healthiest iteration of any type of relationship is when one person lovingly supports and cares for another while each person tends to the inner work that keeps them stuck, hurt, and limited. It is easier to orient yourself toward a loved one from this perspective while you are embodied in true Self. Remember, in true Self you remain clear about the interpersonal boundaries and individual responsibilities that are necessary for healthy relationship participants to thrive together and nourish one another.

Parts Work in Parenting

It might be easy to wrap your mind around allowing adults to be adults with all of their dysfunctional parts in tow without jumping in to rescue them, but what about when you are the parent of a child who is obviously struggling? The limits and boundaries are different, for sure, but essentially the same rules apply. At the core of a healthy parent-child relationship is the dignity that grants your child the right to their own thoughts, feelings, reactions, and responses. This includes standing by as a supportive presence while your child's experiences kick them in the teeth every once in a while. Let's be honest, despite your best intentions you're probably going to wound your child in some way. You likely won't intend to, but you will. We all will. Any parent who believes that they will raise a child with no issues, traumas, or struggles is greatly mistaken and needs a reality check. We live in a complex world with many factors, and it's not possible to get through it without ruffling a few feathers. Your children might be impacted negatively by you, their friends or teachers, or unforeseen accidents and life circumstances. It is not important that your child lives a scathe-free childhood. It is important that they have a sturdy bond with you, their mature adult caregiver who is reliably grounded in true Self (at least most of the time).

Just like your parts can clash with those of your friends and romantic partners, you may also have young unhealed parts that rise to the surface in response to your children. In fact, your children are more likely than anyone else to trigger certain unhealed parts within you because the quality of a parent-child bond allows for incredibly deep vulnerability and intimacy. It's hard to hide much of anything when you are so profoundly connected to a person—and that's okay, it comes with the job. When your defiant twelve-year-old evokes an aggressive part of you that demands respect, try to notice the interplay at hand—even if you can do so only in hindsight once the flames recede. Your child's behavior brought you face to face with a part of yourself (let's call it The Aggressor) that learned to use aggression to secure respect in order to keep you safe in uncertain circumstances. Of course it's not acceptable to act with hostility toward your child, but it can be a powerful learning opportunity if you allow it to be. Once you understand the function of The Aggressor, you can bring that material to your therapy sessions or inner reflective process and heal it. Then down the road when your child behaves defiantly again (as they're oh so likely to do) you will relate from a more healed and grounded place from which you can respond rather than react. Your awareness, healing, and integration of The Aggressor will likely facilitate a more effective solution to work with your child rather than flying off the handle in ways you may later regret.

Another way your children can unintentionally activate your unhealed parts is when one of your wounded child parts envies the healthier, safer, or more stable reality of your child's experience that you did not get to enjoy as a child. This can happen when your child behaves in ways you felt too unsafe to embody in your own childhood. Your unhealed parts might remember being harshly punished, rejected, or emotionally exiled for simply acting like a child—being messy, making annoying sounds, refusing to clean your room, and so on—and you knowingly or unknowingly bring the unhealed trauma of these experiences into parenting your own children. When this happens, you might hear yourself saying things like "I was never allowed to behave like that" or "I wouldn't dream of doing such a thing in my father's house." Such insights allow you to see how much different (and safer) your children's childhood is from your own, and this can be both uncomfortable and reinforcing to experience—even in adulthood. You can work on cultivating self-compassion for your unhealed wounds and motivate to heal them while also feeling proud of the positive intentions you sustained in adulthood to create a healthier world for your descendants.

> **How-To Tip**   If you are a parent, journal about what parts your children evoke in you. It may take a while to gain insight into this topic if you have not yet explored the wounds you carry related to parenting or childhood envy, so please be patient with yourself. It may be helpful to find old photographs of yourself at different times in childhood, maybe at the ages of your current children, and stretch your memory to imagine the thoughts, feelings, and experiences of those younger versions of yourself. Then in your journal ask the parts of you from your photographs how they feel about your current children, your role as a parent, and anything else they wish to share with you. Try to remain open to whatever flows through your writing. You might be surprised by what surfaces.

Practicing parts work in your self-reflective process around parenting and close relationships can provide many fruitful highlights for your inner growth. You might gain awareness about specific parts that get triggered by the oppositional parts of another person in your life, or learn that it is possible for your parts to be gently witnessed by a safe loved one. You may also come to discover that you can place your parts in the light of your own observation (maybe for the first time) and work with them to access potent levels of healing. It is undeniable that your parts are constantly interfacing with those of your friends, family members, colleagues, neighbors, and all other fellow humans you cross paths with. Take it gently as you learn to orient yourself toward yours and other people's parts from a true Self perspective. If this topic lights you up, check out Dr. Richard Schwartz's work and explore his powerful teachings about Internal Family Systems therapy for a deeper dive.

CHAPTER 9

Trauma and Trust

From Friendships to Family to the Shamans of Africa

Trust and safety are the peanut butter and jelly of a relationship. The depth of trust between two people reveals the extent to which they can be themselves together, allow one another freedom and autonomy, and explore their respective lives in tandem without the stifling energetics of suspicion or hypervigilance. I often think of two people in a relationship like two trees growing together. In an ideal situation, the trees (people) grow side by side, providing one another with enough space to expand and branch out while also remaining connected by a strong root system. If the trees grow into each other, they can suffocate one another, get cut off from the sunshine, and limit each other's growth. I see trust as one of the main indicators of whether the two trees of a human relationship grow together, apart, or unhealthfully tangled in knots.

Even within the dyad of a tight mother-daughter bond, a committed partnership, or the most intimate friendship, two people will always remain two separate individuals. When I work with family members or couples who present like a symbiotic organism—behaving as one enmeshed unit rather than two separate beings with individual wants, needs, perspectives, and experiences—I know we've got some good work ahead of us. Clients like these must learn to extract themselves from one another and reclaim the uniqueness of their individual Selves. When they discover a healthy coexistence as two separate beings with individual views and cadences, I know there has been growth. Like a Venn diagram, each person is their own circle, and the overlapping center point between the two circles is where the relationship exists. This middle section is also where relational trust lives. Depending on the degree of trust between two people, their respective individual circles will contain the ripples of those energetics.

> **How-To Tip**   On a large piece of paper, draw a Venn diagram displaying the dynamics between yourself and someone you feel close to. In your and their circles, draw symbols or use collage imagery and words to represent what makes each of you unique and individual. In the overlapping section between your circles, use symbols, images, and words to represent your shared values, beliefs, experiences, connections, and memories.

Dynamics with strong degrees of trust will allow for individuals to feel freedom, sovereignty, and personal agency both when they spend time together and when they are apart. A person in a trusting bond like this feels safe within the steady structure of the relationship and lives without fear of what their behaviors will incite in the other. In a dynamic with weak trust, however, participants often feel strain or pressure when spending time together or apart. They may feel the need to shut themselves down or close themselves off emotionally in order to preserve harmony in their fragile bond. Mistrust stunts a person's growth, autonomy, and independence because they forsake important personal qualities by self-sacrificing in a dynamic that lacks trust.

Ideally, all relationships would have strong and satisfying degrees of trust, but we know from living life in the twenty-first century that this is not always the case. Rather than judging yourself, your counterpart, or your relationship for its imperfect trust dynamic, consider these four options. They will guide you to productively work with your relationship and discern whether the trust level can be improved or not, and what to do if mistrust cannot be amended:

1. *Repair*: If a relationship lacks trust and both parties involved are committed to doing the personal and joint work to heal the rupture that caused the breach, the relationship can regain a healthy level of trust to continue onward.

2. *Learning*: If both parties acknowledge a breach of trust in the relationship and either it cannot be repaired or the people involved are not willing to put in the work to repair it, the relationship can end while serving as a valuable learning experience.

3. *Demise*: If one person feels untrusting while the other refuses to acknowledge and learn about their counterpart's experience with compassion and curiosity, the rupture will remain as long as denial and avoidance dominate the dynamic. In most cases, this foreshadows the relationship's demise.

4. *Intimacy*: Different types of relationships can exist with varying degrees of trust intact. For some, full and complete trust is necessary for safety and security. For other relationships, trust is less important than other factors. Let's explore this option in greater detail.

I do not need the same degree of trust from an acquaintance I enjoy an occasional cup of coffee with as I do from my husband. If my acquaintance is flakey, judgmental, or gossipy, I will not be wounded to the extent that the same offenses from my husband would incite. Why? Because I expect far less from ac-quaintances than I do from my committed life partner. I can un-derstand the degree of trust (or lack thereof) between myself and an acquaintance, adjust my expectations to suit the dy-namic, and remove pressure for that peripheral relationship to sustain me in a meaningful way. Does this mean we can't enjoy coffee together periodically? Absolutely not. It simply means that I will intentionally steer our conversations toward lighter topics rather than seeking emotional support and divulging my secrets and insecurities. I don't need to end a relationship with someone I cannot plummet to the depths of intimacy with— unless, of course, the relationship is unhealthy. I only need to recognize the value of that lighthearted connection and accept it for the good it brings to my life.

Just as we have many different kinds of relationships, there are also varying degrees of trust that may be healthy in those connections. I am thankful to not need deep trust and security with my yoga teacher, a grouchy neighbor, or the PTA crew from my children's school. It releases immense pressure to allow most of my relationships to exist somewhere in the fluid range of trust and be highly discerning about whom I expect greater trust and intimacy from.

While some relationships require less trust than others and can healthfully exist wherever they land on the continuum, others demand deep trust in order to serve a person's highest good. It can be confusing (and heartbreaking) when a relation-ship's trust compass changes midway through the dynamic, when a relationship that was once trustworthy encounters a shift that derails its participants from the rhythm they need to feel safe and secure with one another. Betrayal can act as a dis-ruptor of this kind.

Betrayal

Betrayal creates a break between individuals that can be felt down to the core depending on its circumstances and outcome. When one person feels betrayed by another, it most likely means that their expectations of the sanctity of the relationship's verbal or nonverbal agreements have been dishonored. Betrayal covers a lot of ground and can look differently depending on the dynamic. It ranges from sexual or emotional infidelity within partnerships to gossiping behind a friend's back, from revealing a person's valuable secret to omitting important information in communication. It can be irreparably damaging when you believe you can trust someone, place your heart in their hands, and then feel betrayed by that person's treatment of your sacred vulnerability. Experiences like this can lead you to the *mend* or *move on* choice point where you begin to question whether the relationship is worth continuing or if you would be safer and freer without the hypervigilance required to remain connected to someone you no longer trust.

Sometimes betrayal results from pure thoughtlessness, and other times it can be a calculated plan based on vengeance or cruelty. Regardless of its type, betrayal is a deeply painful experience. In reaction to hurtful disloyalty, a person can spiral in shame for allowing themselves to trust another, shut down their heart for fear of future betrayal, or develop overarching core beliefs about relationships being inherently unsafe based on the wound they acquired.

John Gottman, a world-famous couples therapist, developed the concept of *the four horsemen*[1] to illustrate how people most often betray one another with four common relational patterns: criticism, contempt, defensiveness, and stonewalling. These problematic behaviors have been found in Gottman's research to be wildly destructive to the health, stability, and longevity of relationships, which is why he compares them to the Four Horsemen of the Apocalypse that indicate the end of days in the New Testament. Though it may seem dramatic, there is a good reason for Gottman's identification of the four horsemen. When people in relational dynamics heal these detrimental behavioral impulses, the quality of their bond strengthens and rejuvenates for lasting satisfaction. To break it down into more detail, here are my definitions for each of Gottman's four horsemen:

1. *Criticism*: Different from offering constructive feedback or voicing a complaint about specific issues, criticism is an attack on another person's character.

2. *Contempt*: Contempt involves communication, both verbally and nonverbally, that is truly cruel. When a person treats another with sarcasm, name-calling, minimizing, ridiculing, or using rude body language (such as eye-rolling) they are using contempt. This behavior aims to make a person feel worthless, despised, humiliated, and insignificant.

3. *Defensiveness*: Typically in response to criticism, defensiveness is a behavior that instates one person's innocence or victimization without the willingness to take responsibility for their actions or accountability for their mistakes.

4. *Stonewalling*: This behavior occurs when one person withdraws from another by shutting down, not responding, or zoning out. It also happens when someone starts scrolling through social media while their partner is speaking to them. Stonewalling is a harmful and evasive behavior that dodges conflict by means of disconnecting.

> **How-To Tip** Draw Gottman's four horsemen, metaphorically representing their different qualities. For example, the "stonewalling" horseman might be holding his cell phone in front of his face to represent his inaccessibility to connection. The "criticism" horseman might have six hands with all fingers pointing judgmentally toward others. For further processing, journal about your image and what it means to you.

Becoming aware of Gottman's four horsemen and consciously avoiding the use of such behaviors in relational dynamics is a strong first step toward healing painful interpersonal discord and conflict. Remember, betrayal exists on a continuum of severity. Even the smallest offense can be perceived differently by the person who receives it from what was originally intended. Disloyalty, infidelity, and lack of availability are only some of the ways such an experience can present, and another important trust violation occurs from relational trauma.

Trauma: The Ultimate Breach of Trust

My simplest definition of *trauma* is this: Trauma is when something happens to you, large or small, that derails your feeling of safety in your body, mind, relationships, or world. It messes with your trust in yourself, others, or your larger experience. Trauma is an experience, or set of experiences, that signals danger to your brain and nervous system. Whether the danger is real, perceived, or imagined is irrelevant. Your belief that you are unsafe overrides any cognitive reasoning that you might be mistaken or overreacting. You simply respond from a primal stance of survival in the moment. When your system engages its high-alert reaction and activates the mode where it will do anything to defend itself, nothing is off the table. This is where fight, flight, freeze, and fawn come in. When you feel threatened you will engage any and all capacities to regain safety—whether that means running away, preparing for battle, shutting down, people-pleasing, or pretending to be an entirely different person from the one you are.

My favorite model of how trauma is processed by the nervous system is polyvagal theory, which was developed by Dr. Stephen Porges.[2] This section gets a little technical, so if you're not on board feel free to skip forward. Polyvagal theory is centered around the *vagus nerve*, which is a cranial nerve that plays a major role in soothing the nervous system. By regulating the *parasympathetic nervous system*, essentially the brakes of the nervous system, the vagus nerve helps us calm and soothe ourselves. In counterbalance to the *parasympathetic* is the *sympathetic nervous system*, which is our hub for fight and flight. This system gets activated when the mind and body perceive danger and feel compelled to protect, defend, and survive. When a person is in a calm yet active state of focus, learning, and presence, this nervous system state is called *ventral vagal activation*. This is a healthy mode to be in, a regulated state where you feel safe, stable, and capable of moving effectively through your world.

The various stimuli and impacts of human life make it impossible to exist permanently in ventral vagal activation—so overachievers, manage your expectations. Think of ventral vagal as your healthy home base, a regulated state you aim to return to after fluxing and flowing with the adaptive nature of the nervous system. In anxiety or tension, you will elevate into *sympathetic activation*, and it is also possible during dysregulation that you may drop into *dorsal vagal activation*. This is a shutdown, collapse, "play dead" nervous system response that activates when your system gets overwhelmed and discerns that running away and fighting will not work, so playing dead is the last-ditch effort for survival. In *dorsal vagal activation* a person feels lethargic, heavy, disconnected, and hopeless. More excessive than the gentle brakes of a toned parasympathetic response, dorsal vagal activation is an abrupt slam and hold of the brake pedal where you come to a screeching stop.

Both sympathetic activation and dorsal vagal activation are possible responses when a person's mind, body, and/or heart become dysregulated during traumatic or impactful life events. The good news is that vacillation between nervous system states is not problematic; it is expected in a normal healthy human. It's actually what you're built for. It is when a person gets stuck for a prolonged period of time in either sympathetic or dorsal vagal activation that their system becomes unhealthy. Too much time spent in sympathetic activation can lead to chronic anxiety, high blood pressure, insomnia, impulsivity, and hypertension. Stuckness in dorsal vagal activation can lead to major depression, severe exhaustion, dissociation, and apathy toward relationships and experiences. *Ventral vagal activation* is the sweet spot between the two survival extremes. It is a neutral base from which you can ramp up and down but always return to stability and regulation.

Fawning is a nervous system survival state that is not often talked about, or at least it gets much less press than the ever-popular *fight*, *flight*, and *freeze*—and it's all about trust. When your nervous system shifts into a tense, alert state of sympathetic activation that believes the only way to survive is to keep anyone who seems to be a threat happy, you're fawning. This is where compliance, placating, and people pleasing behaviors are utilized in a desperate attempt to play nice with someone who seems dangerous. On a deep level, your nervous system doesn't trust that you will be safe with the other person unless you comply with them entirely. You may not trust them, the situation, or yourself in their presence—and this can be conscious or unconscious. When effective, fawning manipulates the threatening person to back down, which then returns your nervous system to an experience of safety. *Fawning* can mask as kindness in a charged and stressful relationship dynamic, but when closely inspected for flaws it becomes obvious that it is an adaptive mechanism for protection that has likely become a well-worn pattern over the years.

A person who habituates to fawning during interpersonal stress might regularly tolerate harmful and damaging treatment from others in order to *keep the peace* or *not rock the boat*. No matter what you tell yourself in a moment of justification, fawning does not develop trust. You cannot make an unsafe relationship safe by complying with its dysfunction. You are not in a healthy relationship if the other person is the only one who feels peaceful and you feel untrusting, resentful, abused, or taken advantage of. Fawners, read that last sentence again. A truly peaceful dynamic involves nonviolent nervous system regulation for all involved, not just the person in dominant power. Fawning to ensure another person's peace while simultaneously abandoning your own is one manifestation of how your nervous system protects you in a moment of interpersonal threat—but make no mistake, it is not a solid long-term solution. A momentary survival strategy to regain safety when exposed to a dangerous person is not meant to be a persistent relational dynamic. When you sustain an ongoing position of peacekeeping and compliance in your relationships at the expense of your own peace, your body marinates in stress hormones that inwardly confirm the fear that you are not (and may never be) safe unless you give away your personal power. To break free from an automatic survival response like fawning, you must link your people pleasing behaviors with your nervous system awareness. With deeper self-reflection and inner discovery, you will learn

that what once seemed kind and agreeable is actually a sophisticated response to threat.

You may recognize that you have a default setting when it
comes to how your nervous system reacts when you get dysregulated. Oftentimes people report that they commonly experience the high stimulation state of anxiety or the low state of
depression when the going gets rough. I had always defaulted
to high-stim sympathetic activation when life threw me curve-
balls, but during one particularly difficult time in life my system uncharacteristically explored the terrain of dorsal vagal
activation for the first time.

In my mid-thirties I made the impactful choice to go no-
contact with an abusive family member I had been relationally
miserable with for decades prior. It took many years of inner
work and healing to reach the level of self-confidence and clarity I needed to finally walk away from my abuser, and I did.
Around the same time, I was diagnosed with a relatively common and treatable form of cancer, for which I promptly underwent invasive surgery. The combination of my emotional and
physical experiences at that time culminated in a resulting exhaustion, emotional disconnection, and fogginess that I had
never before experienced. Not until I had been swimming in the
shadows of my surgical recovery and emotional tenderness for
weeks did it occur to me that I had dropped into dorsal vagal
activation. For the first time in my life, I experienced the lows
of dorsal vagal dysregulation rather than the zings of sympathetic activation. Once I understood what was happening, I
cared for myself in a compassionate, loving way that honored
my nervous system's unfamiliar experience. I nurtured myself
back to ventral vagal activation where I felt calm yet energized,
emotionally stable, and much more like myself again. It took
time to buoy myself back to a state of regulation where my sleep,

physical energy level, and interpersonal capacity functioned normally, but I did recover. My relational trauma combined with my cancer experience had me stuck in a down-regulated nervous system state that was wildly foreign to my cognitive understanding. Dorsal vagal activation kept me frozen in a self-perception of danger until I regained the bandwidth and capacity to find my footing again.

Now that you understand the polyvagal perspective of how trauma affects the nervous system, let's look more closely at trauma itself. A physical trauma is an experience where something happens to your body that requires your system to drop whatever functions it's attending to and focus exclusively on the damage that has ensued from a triage perspective—*all hands on deck!* Your pupils dilate, heart rate increases, senses sharpen, and awareness narrows. This happens in response to emotional trauma as well, but it can be less obvious than physical trauma because there may not be blood or broken bones to provide physical evidence of the injury that occurred. For this reason, psychological and emotional trauma can be complex and confusing to pin down. Human beings tend to perceive what they can see with their eyes as being *real* and question the rest as being *make believe* or *imagined*. For this reason, the diagnosis and treatment of emotional and psychological trauma often requires the clinical skillset of a licensed mental health professional to bring invisible pain and suffering to the light for processing, understanding, and ultimately healing. Although trauma exists in countless shapes and forms, for the purpose of this book I will speak to the phenomenon of *relational trauma*: trauma that results from abuse, misalignment, cruelty, and harm within relationships.

To organize terms, therapists and psychologists often refer to *big T* and *little t* traumas as the two general buckets where trauma exists. *Big T* traumas are mostly thought of as the indisputable moments of impact or injury that cause undeniable harm to a person—events like the sudden tragic death of a loved one, rape, school shootings, and other horrific events that can be pinpointed to a certain date and likely attracted immediate help and attention.

Little t traumas, on the other hand, are much more challenging to locate, pin down, and even reach general consensus on regarding their traumatic nature. These are the painful experiences we live through that don't make a huge splash for all to see but nonetheless inflict a discernable slash across our hearts and psyches. Such traumas, often invisible, are frequently exacerbated by repetition, denial, minimization, or disbelief. *Little t* traumas can look like ongoing emotional or verbal abuse, defamation of character, a deeply troublesome interaction (or series of interactions), a personal failure, or an identity or self-worth wound. The saying *death by a thousand papercuts* accurately captures the distress of relational *little t* traumas that repeat and build up over time. *Microaggressions* are repetitive harmful interactions between people, little attacks that accumulate in size, intensity, and impact over time. As microaggressions stack up, they corrode a person's self-worth, intrinsic value, and belief in their lovability.

One example is Adam and Shane's slow-simmering abusive relationship. In a quest for control and power, Adam repeatedly utilized punitive cruelty, harmful words, and/or psychological weaponry in the forms of gaslighting and other manipulation tactics. He belittled Shane's opinions if they differed from his own, attacked his vulnerabilities, and slandered him to their mutual loved ones. Shane knew, on some level, that Adam's cutting words and mind games were unhealthy, but it was difficult for Shane to confront Adam because each small attack was crafted with such subtly. Nothing ever seemed significant enough to hold on to. Eventually, through therapy, Shane learned about microaggressions and everything changed. He recognized the buildup of attacks that had previously seemed like innocent moments of discord. Shane ultimately learned to walk away from his abusive relationship with Adam, rejecting the dynamic that regularly undermined his self-worth. It's possible that a person might easily recover from one or two isolated experiences of relational trauma, but exposure over years or decades like Shane's piles up to create an undeniable wound.

Relational trauma occurs as a result of the things we *do* to each other (overt harm, abuse, humiliation) as well as the things we *don't do* that the other truly needs (attunement, connection, attention, care). This is where neglect and abandonment come in. In some situations neglect can be equally (or even wildly more) damaging than the harm created by intrusive violence. As exclaimed in an episode of *Cheers* in the '90s as well as more recently in a Lumineers song, the opposite of *love* might actually be *indifference*. To feel as though an important person in your life does not care about you, or in extreme cases believes they would be better off without you, develops a trauma response that sits like dry ice in the center of your heart. It can make you question the value of your very existence both physically and existentially. When indifference is prolonged and continuous, a person can develop core beliefs about themselves based on their perceived unworthiness that spider into every one of their relationships and life interactions.

Trauma: How, When, and to Whom

There is a lot of buzz these days about childhood trauma and inner child healing, which is unquestionably a valuable area for inner work. When traumatic experiences happen to a child, the damage is profound and unspeakable. The wounds that accrue in an innocent child's developing psyche are among the deepest and most ingrained roots of many issues people face later as adults. Certainly, much trauma inflicted upon children is intentional and overtly abusive. Additionally, there are forms of trauma young children accrue from well-intentioned caregivers who mean their child no harm, yet damage ensues regardless.

Childhood trauma education and resources are so accessible and thought-provoking that a person might forget that trauma can happen at any age. I have worked with many clients who insist that their childhood was healthy and trauma-free, yet they remain puzzled by the undeniable trauma responses they feel toward their early caregivers and present-day connections. They also may notice intrinsic relational patterns or negative identifications with the Self that they cannot find an origin for in childhood. It is entirely possible for these individuals that their trauma happened outside the bubble of childhood where so many people wrongly assume all wounds originate. It needs to be said: Trauma is trauma at any developmental stage. Adolescent and adult trauma are as legitimate and valid as those from childhood.

In my healing journey, I discovered that the majority of my overt relational trauma from my biological family began when I left home at eighteen to go to college. From that point on, it persisted for decades. As any therapist will tell you, trauma doesn't just appear out of nowhere. In the years before my escape to college, I persevered throughout my childhood in a suspended state of hypervigilance and compliance to avoid evoking what I sensed would be a catastrophic waterfall of abandonment and abuse if I stepped a toe out of line. I call this the *sleeping giants awareness of childhood.* This is when a child senses that they are in danger, so they do everything in their power to tiptoe around their caregivers to avoid awakening the terrifying response they fear lies just beneath the surface. In my mind, I imagine an overall-clad, pigtailed little one precariously navigating a grassy field that is riddled with the monstrous bodies of vengeful, snoring giants she fears awakening.

> **How-To Tip**   Visualize, draw, or write about how you imagine the sleeping giants. Are they huge? Ugly? Drooling? Do they have weapons? Maybe one giant sleeps with an eye open so you must avoid its line of sight for safety. Be imaginative and consider including your young Self. Is your inner child's face fearful? Disconnected? Energized? Maybe they tiptoe carefully, or maybe they hold a shield and pepper spray for protection. Your inner child may be alone, or maybe they have a guard dog, protective adult, or spiritual figure with them.

Commonly, when someone in adulthood shares their psychological and emotional pain with childhood caregivers in an attempt at repair, they are met with utter bafflement and denial. Often, caregivers cannot accept that you harbor wounds inflicted by them because they remember your childhood only as privileged and happy from their avoidant perspective. Their denial and dismissiveness of your *little t* traumas make it nearly impossible to heal these relationships. Long, painful journeys of toxicity often ensue in the wake of a caregiver's unwillingness to see your pain as valid because it wasn't inflicted by monsters they associate with being "abusers" like axe murderers and rapists (perpetrators of big T trauma).

When someone refuses accountability for the role they played in another's pain, as their parent or in any other type of relationship, they isolate the wounded person in their experience and abandon them in the repair alone. This profoundly damages trust between individuals and can catapult a relationship into *mend* or *move on* territory where they are unsure if they should continue holding on to the connection. In many cases like this, it is healthier to *move on* than remain bonded to someone who perpetuates narratives that place you in the scapegoat or villain role to preserve their perception that they are innocent or victimized rather than a cocreator of the dynamic. A person who has endured painful experiences needs to be seen in their experiences and told *I believe you*—especially from people they are supposedly closely bonded with. Though seemingly trivial, those three little words—*I believe you*—have the power to move mountains when it comes to relationship repair. Especially for someone who has experienced the invisible trauma of psychological and emotional abuse, when their pain is seen as valid it affirms their very humanity and communicates to their heart that they are valuable, important, and deserving of love.

Even if trust has been lost within a relationship because of one person knowingly or unknowingly harming another, it can and will be robustly strengthened when both parties willingly acknowledge the pain. It might take layers of healing for a relationship to be restored to a degree of health and intimacy that may or may not have previously existed in the dynamic, so be patient. It is important to understand that trusting, safe relationships are built through continuity and repetition over time. Whatever energetics exist on repeat between two people will build psycho-emotional responses within both parties akin to the frequency of the ongoing dynamic. When conscious intention is thoughtfully wielded to develop relationships of genuine love and stability, robust and radiant connections are made.

Secrets

One phenomenon that can massively rupture trust between people is secret keeping. According to Columbia University research conducted by Michael L. Slepian,[3] 97 percent of people harbor at least one secret at any given time, with the average person actively concealing more or less a dozen secrets. Of these dozen, most people admit to having five secrets they have never told even a single person. Furthermore, Slepian and his researchers identified thirty-eight specific categories of secrets that people commonly keep. These range from illegal behavior to pregnancy, from infidelity to planned surprises for other people (like surprise birthday parties), and many others.[4] Slepian's research suggests that we all keep the same kinds of secrets, but why? How is it beneficial for the human psyche to conceal and keep things to ourselves? As it turns out, there are two main reasons that make perfect sense:

1. We are afraid that people will judge *our secrets* as wrong or bad.

2. We are afraid that people will judge *us* as wrong or bad for hiding our secrets.

> **How-To Tip**   Are you thinking about your secrets? Good! Take a moment to journal about what this brings to the surface for you.

All suffering related to secret keeping comes down to the avoidance of feeling *wrong* or *bad*. This tracks with our human needs for love and belonging in relationships and our desire to preserve our image in the eyes of others as being *good* or *right*. The truth, as proven by Slepian's research, is that most everyone keeps secrets. So it's less about the behavior itself and more about the longevity of the behavior that indicates the possible negative impacts a secret can have. The longer a secret remains hidden, the bigger the consequences from its hiding may be. When a person keeps a secret for a long time, fear #2 (that people will judge us as wrong or bad for hiding the secret) grows in like-liness and accumulates significant stress. When a person keeps a secret, their mind wanders to the secret far more frequently than the requirement to actively conceal the secret requires. It can be assumed that the longer this process persists, the more intensity builds surrounding continuous revisitation of the stressor. When it comes to the negative effects of secret keep-ing, it is the frequency at which a person thinks about the secret that most harms their well-being rather than the concealment itself. As Slepian and his researchers delved one thousand people and six thousand secrets deeper into their data, they discovered that the types of secrets people dwell on most frequently, thus impacting the most profoundly negative impacts on them-selves, are secrets they feel ashamed of rather than those they feel guilty about.[5]

Though shame and guilt are often coupled together as simi-lar emotions, meaningful differences set them apart. *Guilt* relates to feeling badly about something you have done. It is adaptive in the sense that when you feel guilty, you feel somehow capa-ble of making amends or finding a takeaway from the experi-ence that impacts improved future behavior. *Shame*, however, relates to feeling as though it's not your behavior that was wrong but your Self. You feel like a bad or harmful person con-sumed by a helplessness to ever change yourself to be better. It is this particular powerlessness over the quality of Self-goodness that can create a loop within a person that leads them to repeat-edly revisit their shameful secrets and suffer the negative consequences.

It might seem obvious that secret keeping disrupts the deli-cate balance of trust within a relationship, but if 97 percent of people are keeping secrets at any given time, you can easily as-sume that such breaches exist in even the happiest and healthiest of relationships. Sure, many people may be blissfully unaware that their best friend, boss, or significant other is keeping a secret from them, but it might also be true that the secret holds little weight over what truly matters in the connection. For example, when Drea keeps the secret from her partner that she has been swapping out her daily exercise routine for an office happy hour, it likely matters much less than when Abe kept the secret of a three-month-long sexual affair from his romantic partner. In another example, Telly's secret use of her colleague's pencil collection is likely insignificant compared to her secretive sharing of sensitive computer data without her company's explicit permission to do so. The two things that matter most about secrecy are the magnitude and longevity of a secret and a person's degree of shame regarding what they did.

As anyone who has ever harbored a burning secret knows, those slippery suckers tend to find their way into the light despite our Herculean efforts to conceal them. Be it because of carelessness, a misstep in strategically laid lies, or the blatant exhaustion involved with the prolonged concealment of a shameful secret, the things we hope to keep to ourselves forever tend to get revealed eventually. This is when the trust between people gets thrust upon the relational chopping block.

When a long-held secret gets revealed (or even a short-held one, for that matter), it exposes an area within a relationship where there was likely a preexisting wound or fissure that already impacted instability in the dynamic. If there were only strength and trust to be found in the connection, there would be no need for secret keeping. So it is the responsibility of the people involved in a relationship where a secret is revealed to discern together what factors caused the lack of honesty, whether the rupture can be mended, and what is necessary to foster a successful repair.

If the parties involved can perceive the secret as an opportunity to strengthen their bond by working on the relationship's weak spots, they have a pretty solid chance for double-strengthened dynamics in the future. Such reinforcement is built from the process of rupture and repair fostered by the secret and its subsequent integration with honest effort between kindred souls who choose to observe it together. Similar to the surgical repair of a torn ligament or tendon with a graft from elsewhere in the body, when a relational rupture is met with intentional bolstering that stitches it carefully back together, it becomes stronger than ever before. Conversely, if a rupture is met with avoidance, denial, carelessness, or apathy, it can only remain frayed and broken. Situations like these are common in relationships that were already suffering and teetering on the verge of collapse or those with covert issues that the participants had been consciously or unconsciously unwilling to rectify. This is why in some relationships a person seeks out an instigator to effectively end a relationship they already want out of but are unsure how to escape, like a romantic relationship participant pursuing an affair.

If a person is motivated enough that they are willing to engage the healing necessary to mend a wound that was caused by secret keeping or any other issue, there's a great deal of hope for a successful repair. Conversely, if someone's unhappiness is central and they lack the intention for interpersonal healing, the end of the relationship is likely imminent. When a person feels remorse and regret that ultimately leans them closer toward the relationship, recognizing its value and fighting for its continuation, good things can happen. This is where the difficult territory of apologies and forgiveness comes in.

Apologies and Forgiveness

The single most important thing to know about apologies and forgiveness is this: An apology does not guarantee forgiveness. Hard stop. I'll repeat this for those of you in the back: Just because you apologized, even if it was the most stellar heartfelt apology imaginable, you are not guaranteed forgiveness immediately or ever. An apology is the responsibility of the person who caused harm, and forgiveness is not theirs to determine. The person who was hurt has complete and total control over if, when, how, and with what conditions they chose to offer forgiveness. Sometimes a meaningful apology suffices to unlock a person's genuine forgiveness. In other cases, forgiveness evolves over time with proof that the wrongdoer feels true remorse for the pain they inflicted. Sometimes a person never reaches forgiveness at all. None of these options is up to the apologizer. It's the way energetics flow, frustrating as it may be to exist solemnly on the sending end of an apology without knowing how it is being received and what the outcome will be. This is one of life's great lessons that can be difficult to swallow—especially for someone who feels genuine remorse and regret. The person's degree of patience, however, while their loved one determines their route toward forgiveness, is their choice. It's usually fruitless to try to force a person to stick around if they don't want to. And at the end of the day, regardless of whether they receive forgiveness or not, the offender may be unwilling to wait for the forgiver's acceptance of their amends. They might simply be done.

Forgiveness can be a particularly bitter pill to swallow for many people because of the special blend of humility, accountability, and remorse it necessitates. It requires a person to take a wide-lens perspective toward someone who hurt them, which can be tough when you're in pain. Let's be honest, compassionate understanding can be difficult to drum up amid hurt feelings and betrayal. There's more to forgiveness than meets the eye, though. When a person accesses forgiveness, even partially, they soon discover that forgiveness does not condone the wrongdoing that occurred. Many people incorrectly assume that forgiveness makes the offense that transpired okay, but that's not the higher function of forgiveness at all. At its core, forgiveness relieves a hurt person from carrying an offense inflicted by another in their heart. It allows them to move on, free from the burden of holding grudges and harboring bitterness. Whether they choose to continue the relationship with their offender (*mend*) or not (*move on*) is separate from forgiveness. A person can forgive someone who harmed them while also deciding to end the relationship. In cases where someone decides to *move on*, forgiveness allows them to walk away with dignity and Self-respect, knowing that they took the burden-free higher ground and trusting that releasing grudges frees them to seek healthier relationships as they move away from the detrimental ties of their past. When a person forgives, they let go of anger, resentment, and hatred that had previously fortified their resistance. At the end of the day, forgiveness isn't for the offender. It does not condone their behavior, absolve their sins, or wash clean the injustice of their actions. Forgiveness is for you—for your freedom.

A Jewish Hasidic parable I love tells the story of a rupture between a king and his son. This is how it goes: After being in conflict for some time, the king reached a threshold of rageful impatience and exiled his son from the kingdom. Deeply hurt, the prince left the kingdom to build a life elsewhere. Years passed, and the king's heart softened over time. With the perspective he gained from lengthy time apart from his son, the king yearned for repair. He sent his messengers to find the prince and invite him home to the kingdom. When the messengers finally found the prince, they discovered that he remained deeply wounded from his painful dynamic with his father. In response to their invitation, the prince declined the king's offer. The messengers returned to the kingdom and told the king of his son's continued bitterness and refusal to return. In response, the king sent them to his son once again with a new message: *Return as far as you are able, and I will come the rest of the way to meet you.*[6]

This story beautifully illustrates the delicate relational interplay involved in fostering a genuine, effective repair between people who have been tangled in a difficult dynamic together. Had the king demanded that his son return to the kingdom on the king's terms, without honoring the prince's emotional experience (however inconvenient it may have been), their rupture would have likely persisted, if not grown in magnitude. By attuning to his son's raw emotional wound with softness and promising that he would do anything necessary to heal their relationship, the king displayed genuine remorse and willingness to repair. I remember this touching story when I find myself both asking for forgiveness and being asked for it. It requires a gentle courage to dance within the relational realm of forgiveness and apologies when heated conflict escalates. With the heartfelt example set by the king in the parable, I have found myself able to access the courageous softness that is necessary to navigate this tenuous terrain in multiple areas of my life.

Confusion

It can be challenging to be vulnerable when you feel confused about the quality or integrity of a relationship, and this messes with trust in a deep way. Certain people perceive confusion as mysterious and exciting, an experience where they can incite curiosity. Such a response is healthy and indicates that the person feels safe in the experience of confusion. Sam exemplifies this when he perceives his friend's erratic behavior with curiosity rather than jumping to conclusions about what it means about their relationship. *I wonder why my friend flies off the handle when we talk about his family. There must be more to their relationship than meets the eye.* Other people have a shakier response to feeling confused that indicates feeling unsafe in the experience. This tends to complicate things and put barriers in place that inhibit genuine connection. This happens when confusion arises and someone personalizes, judges, or makes assumptions about the dynamic that could be wildly off base. If Sam were to take this stance, his observation would sound more like *My friend flies off the handle when we talk about his family, so he must have a messed-up family and hate everyone who asks about them.*

For me, confusion has always felt unsafe. Being perpetually gaslit by people I was meant to trust and rely on taught me that when I feel confused, something dangerous is happening in my psyche. In such a state, I have learned from experience to be on high alert and figure out how to urgently regain clarity to ensure my own safety. This pattern is a trauma response that has posed significant problems in my life. When I perceived danger as a child and young adult, I subsequently felt confused, which led me to instinctively live in a highly controlled manner in the cerebral space of my mind. My rigidity served as a lifestyle adaptation I have since worked to repair through years of therapy and inner work with the intention of balancing my nervous system. Though I have grown my tolerance for feeling confused, it still sneaks up on me with red-flag alarms at times.

In adulthood, when I was in a raw layer of healing regarding my family of origin, I found myself following a breadcrumb trail that ultimately led me to work with the shamanic healers of an African tribe. These healers specialize in healing and clearing ancestral wounds for the intergenerational repair of unhealthy patterns throughout a lineage. It took immense courage for me to venture beyond the confines of the Western healing methods I knew and trusted so that I could experience something so wildly different. At the time, I was desperate to try anything.

The method of the particular shamanic work I pursued involved interacting with a woman local to my area for energy work and clearing before she accompanied me as a conduit in cross-continental virtual communication with the African shamans. She introduced me to rituals I would participate in to bring the sacred energy of the African shrine room into my Western home as well as practices to open my nighttime dreamscape to the shamans while they worked remotely with my energy and ancestry. It was all quite foreign and scary for me, but I felt called to trust the process and give it open-mindedness and effort.

Days after I had participated in the prescribed rituals, healing sessions, phone conversations, and subsequent internal and external processing, I was deeply confused by my experience. Somehow I landed on the other side of the experience with many unanswered questions, a great deal of physical and emotional discomfort, and an ongoing perplexity about what had happened and whether it had been effective. I approached the local conduit with questions for which I never received clarity. We seemed to be looking through the same window and seeing incongruent experiences. I aimed to express my inquiries clearly because I wanted to feel understood, and I tried my best to receive her answers with openness because I did not want to be rigid or judgmental. I even prepared a letter of apologetic surrender with the intention of mailing it to the people who had viciously perpetrated against me all my life. I tried so hard to make the experience fit my needs, only to later discover that I had tried too hard. An aligned healing experience shouldn't have a square-peg-round-hole feeling, and this one unmistakably did.

It wasn't until I processed my experience with a trusted mentor that I gained clarity. She helped me understand that my inner system did not feel safe enough to allow me to receive what was being given. I did not feel held in the experience or in the confusion it stirred up, which tanked my trust. Thankfully I spoke to my mentor before I mailed the letter I wrote. I clearly understood in hindsight that its transmission would have undoubtedly reentered me into the scapegoat position I had worked so hard to step out of.

I do not doubt that the wisdom the shamans perceived about my lineage was true and that their work is legitimate and healing. Possibly, I was not ready to receive their healing insight. It is also possible that their flavor of healing was simply not the right flavor for me. Perhaps at a later date the experience will integrate differently and make more sense.

In the landscape of confusion I shared with my mentor, I came to understand something crucial: In order to venture into work such as this, I needed to more deeply heal the internal parts of myself that felt threatened by confusion during times of vulnerability. I learned a valuable lesson: The type of help a person can tolerate and receive during hardship is directly related to the measures of safety they need while the help is being offered. Truly, we cannot absorb something if our doors and pores are closed to it—even if it is the greatest divine medicine of the universe. Systemic safety on all levels (physically, emotionally, cognitively, energetically, and spiritually) is paramount to our ability to heal.

CHAPTER 10

Commitment

When to Keep It, When to Break It

When happiness researcher George Vaillant claimed "Happiness is love. Full stop," his claim was backed by massive research from the longest longitudinal study of human development ever undertaken.[1] Vaillant began the *Grant Study of Adult Development* in 1938, where he studied the physical and emotional health of over two hundred college-age men. These participants were observed through the ages of fifty-five and beyond into their nineties to uncover the truth of what makes people happy through their lifespan. Aspects such as relationships, politics, religion, coping strategies, and alcohol use were all tracked through the years. Overall findings discovered that the single most important trait of happy, healthy elders is—you guessed it—stable, meaningful long-term relationships. Participants who were most satisfied in their relationships at fifty were the healthiest at eighty. In case you're curious, the single greatest disruptor of health and happiness was found to be alcohol abuse.[2]

While researching the greatest enhancers and antagonists of happiness, the Harvard Grant Study clarified that our life choices have a far stronger impact on our satisfaction, fulfillment, and joy than our DNA and genetics do. Welcome to a new level of freedom, my friends, when you realize that you are in control of your own happiness. This means that there's no one to blame but yourself if you feel otherwise.

> **How-To Tip** Create a drawing, painting, or collage of your closest relationships. Consider the setting where you represent these people, and remember to include yourself. Perhaps you might draw a campfire where you and your loved ones gather. If your loved ones live far away, consider drawing yourself in the center of the page with branching spokes that encapsulate and connect you to each meaningful person with lines and shapes. Maybe your closest relationships are apples on the tree that represents your Self. For further processing, write about your creative process and product in your journal.

Whether you have an abundance of intimate familial bonds and few friendships or vice versa, it is imperative that you selectively choose important people to emotionally bond with. Commit intentionally to your connections. Pour your heart, soul, time, and effort into them.

The term "commitment" is often mistaken for long-standing loyalty within a romantic partnership exclusively, but it can (and does) exist in any type of meaningful relationship. Relational commitment simply reflects your intention for dedication and allegiance to another. It is your devotion to ride the waves of emotions and experiences with someone you deem dear. That's where the gold is—in the relationships that have together traversed complex and meaningful territory through the journey of life and remain committed to their bond.

I have a long-standing commitment to my dear friend (I'll call her Claire) that spans nearly two decades at this point. We have both intentionally carved out a two-hour block of time on our calendars to connect every week for all these years. Through rain, snow, pregnancy, trauma, joy, and transition, Claire and I have honored our commitment. When we both lived locally, we met somewhere equidistant from our two neighborhoods. When we lived in different cities, impeccable cell phone reception became crucial for our phone dates. We have seen each other through life. Our commitment is not only strong; it's steadfast and lasting. Though I am no fortune teller and cannot predict the future, I see Claire in my life until the end. The commitment is real, it's mutual, and it has profoundly benefited my happiness and brought meaning to my life.

Whether you express your commitment to your closest people verbally or not, explicitly or not, through marital vows or with loyalty that stands the test of time, an expression of true commitment to an important relationship is a promise that carries great capacity for emotional support. It is akin to the most solid net imaginable. You are genuinely known and seen for who you are, and your counterpart agrees to walk beside you on the gameboard of life. If you have one person like this in your life, or maybe a few (for the lucky ones among us), consider thanking them for their commitment to you. Let these special people know how much you value their love. After all, researchers[3] have discovered that simply saying "thank you" is the single most impactful factor when building strong long-term relationships. Not "I love you" or even "I'm here for you." Just straight-up gratitude is the magical ingredient that helps a relationship thrive for the long, happy haul.

The Window of Tolerance

Though important, gratitude can sometimes feel light-years away, an inconceivable possibility, when you are in conflict with someone. For that reason it is important to build in some wiggle room. One of my favorite tools from dialectical behavior therapy (DBT) is the concept of *the window of tolerance*, which was developed by Dr. Dan Seigel.[4] The window explains the most optimal state of arousal or stimulation a person can experience while remaining able to thrive healthfully in their daily rhythm. Imagine an oceanic body of water with three sections: The topmost section is shallow, the middle section is moderate, and the bottom section is deep and dark. In Seigel's model, the middle section represents the window of tolerance, where a person can feel present, centered, and capable of managing their daily functions with confidence. The shallow section above it represents *hyperarousal*, where a person feels anxious, amped, and flighty. The dark waters of the lowest section represent *hypoarousal*, where a person feels weighted, sluggish, or checked out in apathy and disconnection. In most facets of healthy human life, the goal is not to be hyper or hypo anything, but to be balanced. The window of tolerance reflects this necessity.

When it comes to relational balance, I like using the window of tolerance as a framework to teach about how to achieve healthy connections. If your relationship is in *hyper* territory, you might find yourself overfunctioning, feeling anxious, people pleasing, and buzzing in hypervigilance about how the other person feels about you and what you need to do to keep them happy. *Hypo* territory, on the other hand, feels more like disconnection from the other person, apathy about the state of the relationship, or feeling exhausted by the needs and demands of the dynamic. Like our storybook friend Goldilocks, human systems seek relationships that are neither too *hypo* nor too *hyper* but *just right*. That's the window of tolerance, where you feel nestled safely within a comfortable and safe psycho-emotional zone while also feeling inspired, positively challenged, and meaningfully connected. You may vacillate within the window upward toward *hyper* or downward toward *hypo* during phases or moments when you react to situational experiences, but a healthy relationship remains within the window of tolerance for most of the time.

Often when relationship participants find themselves in a state of compromise, they are deviating from the window of tolerance to some degree. Consider the absolute middle point in the center section as your perfect sweet spot where all the relational stars are beautifully aligned. You're getting everything you want and need from your relationship, giving back feels easy, and your cup is full. It's highly unlikely that you will spend your lifetime in such impeccable alignment all the time—actually, it's impossible. That's why our systems are adaptable and flexible, and a little deviation from the mean is no problem. The temporary escalation toward hyperarousal or sinking toward hypoarousal might look something like these examples:

> *Hyperarousal*: The James family has a vacation coming up. Sally has wanted to get her family packed and ready for days, but her partner, Mila, insists on waiting until the last minute to gather her things. Sally feels a bit anxious and unsettled by the last-minute packing, but she tolerates the distress by allowing Mila to be accountable for her own things while she gets everything else packed up and ready in her preferable timeline. It's not Sally's ideal situation, but it is a compromise her mind and nervous system can tolerate without catapulting into full-on dysregulated *hyper* arousal.

> *Hypoarousal*: It has been a long week for Chris after recovering from the flu and taking care of his kids while they were also sick. Janna never caught the flu and has been looking forward to taking a long family hike over the weekend. When Janna shares her plan with Chris, he expresses exhaustion and unwillingness to be active over the weekend. Janna feels disappointed that she won't be getting the group activity she had

hoped for, but she acknowledges the reality of the situation and brainstorms a pivot that will allow everyone to get what they need without anyone completely leaving their window of tolerance. In Janna's willingness to take it easy while her family recovers from their illness, she might venture out for a shorter hike on her own while the family naps. It's not her ideal, but it's a tolerable compromise.

Neither of the above examples demonstrates the sweet spot of Goldilocks perfection, but the deviations are tolerable and acceptable, if not preferable. These are examples of healthy vacillation within the window of tolerance. If Mila's procrastination becomes pervasive throughout the family dynamic and incites continuous anxiety for Sally, their relationship will meander out of the window and into the *hyper* zone where it will not remain healthy for the long term. If Chris's lethargy and unwillingness to be active become ongoing factors in the family dynamic, Janna will likely feel burdened by his pervasive *hypo* state, and it will not be healthy for them. These examples demonstrate healthy and unhealthy levels of compromise that can determine whether a relationship sinks or floats for the long haul.

> **How-To Tip**   Journal about relationships you have experienced on all three levels of the window of tolerance. Consider how each dynamic worked out for you depending on its degree of relational balance.

If you're taking stock of your relationships and pinpointing their locations on the three-layered map only to discover that you're either *hyper* or *hypo* prone in your connections, you have discovered valuable knowledge to integrate about your relational tendencies. Such an epiphany might explain why you continuously find yourself in repeating patterns with different people. If you notice a cyclical habit like this, explore my book *The Radiant Life Project* to turn this work inward and investigate your core beliefs, narratives, and other influences that keep you looping.

Abandonment vs. Rejection

It is tough to talk about commitment without acknowledging the energetics on the opposite side of the coin: abandonment and rejection. These two words are often used interchangeably to represent the painful experiences of feeling unwanted, unloved, or cast aside by another. Although abandonment and rejection might seem on the surface to encompass similar types of discomfort, they are actually quite different.

When a person is developmentally normal and functions neurotypically, there is no such thing as abandonment in adulthood. There. I said it. Let's break this down, because I can sense the hairs standing up on your arms in denial and rebuttal. The narrative of an abandoned person is usually along the lines of "you left me, so now I will die." Abandonment is a survival response that happens in childhood when a youngster knows on a deep existential level that their very existence depends on being safely connected to their caregivers. In a real way for children, abandonment poses a profound risk to their being. This is because a child has yet to fully develop their personal agency, autonomy, sovereignty, and independence—let alone their brain, which completes development between the ages of twenty-five and thirty. The greatest risk for a child who depends on their caregivers to meet their basic needs is not rejection, where they could experience hurt feelings. Instead, the risk of abandonment reflects the terror of being alone in the world and incapable of meeting their own survival needs.

Once a person has reached developmentally normal adulthood, however, their brain has fully developed. They have acquired the maturity, independence, and autonomy to care for themselves in a reliable, intrinsic way. It's fair to assume that most adults can use the bathroom independently, seek food and feed themselves, form meaningful connections that support their relational needs, and so on. This equates to an adult who has matured to the extent where their inner strength and development make them impossible to abandon. This is because they possess the internal resources to care for themselves without their safety being primally threatened by their reliance on others. When an adult feels cast aside, left behind, or excluded, it is a very real and deeply painful experience of rejection, not the primal experience of abandonment.

Terry Real discusses this distinction.[5] When you understand that *abandonment* is a child's fragile ego state that adults outgrow and rightly label the uncomfortable grief of being cast aside by someone you care about as *rejection*, you regain your personal power. By acknowledging that your safety and survival are not in the hands of anyone except yourself, you reinforce to your inner system that you can capably cultivate and sustain healthy adult relationships where commitment is possible.

When you acknowledge to yourself that your survival is not up for debate because you've got that piece locked in for yourself, you connect and interact with other adults without the dependency a child projects toward their caregiver at an age when abandonment would be so devastating. This frees you to build emotional, heart-centered, and psychologically sound commitments with others. However, as you probably know from experience, it's not always a cakewalk to be in relationships as an adult, even without abandonment as a potential factor. Risks are inherent in the open-hearted vulnerability required by connections of depth and meaning. If you seek a risk-free relationship, you'll have to search on other planets that operate by different laws of relational physics.

One such risk of relational connection that develops when people are mutually committed to each other is (you guessed it) the risk of rejection. Here's where relationship talk gets real, folks. Rejection is always a possibility when individuals begin something together. People change and grow in all kinds of predictable and unpredictable ways, and it is always possible that you might grow apart from someone you once felt impeccably aligned with. Here's the good news for your grown-up brain, nervous system, and psychologically developed adult Self: If the undesirable happens and you do end up feeling rejected by someone you grew to love and interdepend on, you are capable of moving through that experience.

> **How to Tip**   Two journal entries: First, write about a time when you felt rejected. Then write about a time when you rejected someone else. Explore both experiences on physical, emotional, and psychological levels. Note what you learned from each.

If you feel rejected (and I think we all have at some point), please understand that this does not make you in any way *disposable*. Try not to give another person the power to make you feel like you have no value simply because they cannot see it or do not appreciate it. When you are flooded with rejection energy, it can be helpful to remember that the perception someone else brings toward you in a relational dynamic is much more likely to be a reflection of where they're at in their own evolution than having anything to do with you. Let's be honest: Feeling rejected is visceral. So peel your heart from the pit of your stomach. If you feel discarded by someone, it's likely that they are not a good fit for you either. By letting you go, they actively open space in your life for relationships that will be more aligned and resonant for you. Experiment with alchemizing the rejection energy within yourself to clear and open you rather than tarnish and harden you. And always, always, always remember: You are not disposable. You have inherent value as a human being. Go find people who honor and appreciate your gifts, and get in the practice of refusing to dwell on anyone who diminishes your worth.

Commitment Despite Change

It is important to know that it's not a one-way ticket to break-up-ville just because people change throughout their lifespans. In fact, it can be a rich opportunity for the commitment to deepen and access new levels of relational growth.

Here is an example of how this can happen: Deb and Sunny met in college, so by the time they were in their late forties you can imagine how much they had both changed since their nineteen- and twenty-year-old Selves first met. Throughout career changes, pregnancies and parenting, losses, and gains, this couple surfed many of life's waves together. It wasn't until their youngest child entered middle school that Deb and Sunny encountered their first disagreement that monumental challenged their previously rock-solid bond. Sunny reported confusion and feelings of betrayal when seemingly out of nowhere Deb voiced an interest in shifting into a polyamorous dynamic that would provide her with the freedom to date different people while remaining married to Sunny. In expressing her desire,

Deb revealed a part of herself to Sunny that he never knew existed. She was asking her partner to join her in redefining commitment as they knew it and stretch the edges of their marriage in brave new ways. Sunny later told me that this was a "sink or swim" moment for their marriage. He also explained it as "evolve or die" in the sense that he knew his unwillingness to curiously consider the shift Deb required would certainly terminate their relationship. Through a combination of therapy, experimentation, honesty, and clear communication, Deb and Sunny remain married to this day. For them, polyamory served as a catalyst for the individual and relational growth that both parties are now able to reflect on with gratitude.

It's true that not all differing needs through the span of a relationship will unfold with as much compassion and understanding as Deb and Sunny's. Sometimes people grow apart to the extent that they cannot agree on level ground upon which to stand hand in hand anymore—and that's okay. That's what divorce, breakups, estrangement, and thanks-but-no-thanks discernments have in common. Sometimes a relationship simply cannot withstand the change that is required by its members. But not always. In cases where couples, families, friends, or groups are able to pivot together and reinvent their dynamics along the way, certain important ingredients make such evolutions possible. To name a few:

- *Curiosity*: When you can maintain an open mind and consider what you may be missing or possibly don't know about a situation, you open yourself up for learning and growth. Simply approaching a situation with a "tell me more" or "help me understand" mindset can lead to discoveries and insights you may never have experienced otherwise.

- *Softening perfectionism*: Perfectionism is when you are more focused on the granular details that are not working than on the components that are. This is a form of attachment to "perfect" as the best or only route to success, but it is a fallacy. You may have a particular perception of what "perfect" looks or feels like, but by softening your perspective you could discover beauty in the imperfections of your relationships and those you are connected to.
- *Spacious presence*: If you have ever viewed impressionist art, you might recall the differing visual experience between the close-up and far-back views of a painting. Sometimes you're too close to see what is really there; it all looks like a mess of strokes and colors with no definable meaning. Then suddenly, when you take a step or two back, your visual perception converts blobs of shape and color into a picturesque work of art. Sometimes gaining distance from someone or something offers the necessary perspective shift that allows you to effectively understand the whole and bring new appreciation to the up-close details you couldn't previously make meaning of.
- *Nonjudgment*: I'm just going to say it: Who says your way is the right way? Well, besides you, anyway. If you zoom out from your singular vantage point, you might discover that there are many ways to peel a mango. Or skin a cat. Whatever floats your boat. Try to release attachment to your all-knowing ego that thinks your way is the best and only way, and let your judgment recede to open space for learning. There's a whole world out there beyond your perception.

Experiment with considering the validity of opinions, needs, perspectives, and possibilities that before seemed foreign to you.

> **How-To Tip**   Journal about when you either sank or swam when a relationship pivoted from its origin. Note how you felt in this connection. Could you sense the shift happening? Consider how the change felt initially, if the experience shifted over time, and how you feel about it now.

Codependency and Interdependency

Commitment is not the same as codependency, though it can be easy to form a codependent dynamic if a connection is built by two wounded people seeking belonging in the only way they've ever known (although it's dysfunctional). Let's be honest: Who doesn't enter into a friendship, a romantic partnership, or even a business relationship with the best of intentions? I think we can safely assume that most people shoot for *healthy* as their target goal. However, with so many codependent relationships among us, many people clearly shoot and miss (and often by a long shot). This is not a *shoot for the moon, and if you miss at least you'll be among the stars* kind of experience, and I'll tell you why: Once a commitment tumbles toward codependency, it can be challenging to extricate genuine connection from distorted enmeshment. It all comes down to how well a person understands that a relationship comprises two individuals, both with their own lives, who choose to connect without either person abandoning the life that is (and always has been) their own. It's the sometimes confusing nuance of working together in synergy without losing sight of your individuality. This requires that you remain a stable base for yourself while also participating in a duo dynamic that requires your involvement.

It has been seventy-four years since Looney Tunes introduced the cartoon interplay between Wile E. Coyote and the Road Runner,[6] but I'm sure many readers from old-school generations can remember the circles the Road Runner ran around poor Wile E. Coyote that rendered him continuously dizzy. Trying to differentiate the healthy nature of *interdependency* compared to its less beneficial counterpart, *codependency*, can feel a lot like that. Bottom line: You're not looking for codependent relationships but interdependent ones instead. Here are some definitions:

- *Codependency*: Codependency is when you negate a reasonable response or participation in a relationship (like expressing a need) in order to avoid an undesirable outcome (like being shamed for having needs). Even if it seems accommodating, this type of behavior is controlling. It functions to help you sidestep another person's feelings by acting in ways that aim to predict their behavior. This most often happens for the purpose of eliciting certain responses like love and belonging, and avoiding others like anger and rejection. No matter how you slice it, attempting to assert your will to achieve an outcome you desire is always a form of manipulation. I often think of codependency as *I'm only okay if you're okay. Our okayness is inextricably linked, and I do not know where you end and I begin.*
  - *Enmeshment*: Enmeshment is a facet of codependency that can exist between couples, business partners, and friends too, but I will explain it in a parent-child scenario. It is enmeshment when a parent inflates their child's sense of self-esteem

and self-worth, subsequently using them to support their own relational needs. In a situation like this, the support and caregiving flows from the child toward the parent, opposite of how nature intended, which makes the child feel special and important while also feeling deeply responsible (and weary) from the inappropriate pressure inherent in the dynamic. I once had a mentor who explained this type of dynamic as being derailed from "right relationship," where the energy should flow in the direction intended by nature from the parent toward the child—not opposite.

- *Interdependency*: Interdependency is when two conscious adults choose to construct a life, friendship, or partnership while remembering that they are separate beings with their own needs and preferences. It requires recognition that the only person in the relationship you can (and should) control is yourself. From this perspective, you are responsible for showing up in the dynamic with as much accountability and authenticity as possible. This facilitates a healthy relational give-and-take without the burdensome requirement to tiptoe around undesirables.

Basically, *codependency* is reliance based on a perceived need and *interdependency* is reliance based on choice. There is often a great deal of grasping and chasing involved in codependent relationships, as people in such dynamics never feel truly safe. They know, on a deep level, that the connection is conditional and fragile. Bonds like these require that the participants commit entirely to the dysfunctional belief that one person will not be okay without the other, and they will not survive in the wake of the other's disappointment and discontent. Jealousy, mind games, and manipulation can unfold in the shadow of such fears. This only further reinforces the relationship's instability if each person doesn't neatly tuck away their autonomy and play their codependent part.

People who attract codependent dynamics do so for a reason, most often stemming from unhealed relational trauma earlier in life. If you felt abandoned and uncared for in childhood, it makes sense that you might latch on to a person who makes you feel lovable and valuable—even if they do so with the unhealthy conditionality that you must fulfill their needs and desires despite your natural inclination to say no to their demands. Since codependent relationships develop between people who both have healing to do, this type of dynamic functions productively only until one person starts healing what contributes to their participation in the dysfunction. Once a single party grows beyond codependent urges as a result of their inner repair, the codependent dynamic no longer feels snuggly and secure. The other person's dependency on you remaining unhealed functioned for them because it enabled them to do the same. This is why engaging in a healing journey often comes with a lot of goodbyes, both large and small. You may realize that your potent attraction to a certain person (or type of person) in the past now repels you, and you find yourself attracted to an entirely new specimen of human than ever before. This is because along with your healing, you stopped relating to dysfunctional people who fit the mold for the codependency that no longer aligns for you.

You may get sick of hearing about how your adult relationship quality stems from your childhood relational experiences, but in truth that's where your relationships foundation was built. You're attracted to whom you're attracted to for a reason, and it's not always based on healthy desirability. Sometimes your inner system magnetizes toward someone who embodies similar dynamics from relationships of the past that ultimately harmed you. Other times you may feel attracted toward energies you desperately yearned for in childhood but never received. Still other experiences reflect your wounded core beliefs in projection toward another person.

Interpersonal neurobiology studies how our brains and nervous systems are intricately affected by our childhood experiences and ongoing relationships. Early connection impacts our neurobiology in powerful ways as relational adults. The human mind exists in a potent social context that requires connection and co-regulation between different people. Essentially, in relationships we are borrowing and utilizing each other's nervous systems to regulate our own (a phenomenon called *co-regulation*), and we provide that function for each other even if we are unaware that it's happening. The nervous systems, hormone levels, and immune responses of those you are bonded with are directly affected by you, and you reap positive and negative resonance from theirs as well. Modern studies now demonstrate that stable, secure relationships impact a boatload of positive effects in the minds and bodies of all people involved. This includes increased immunity, physical and mental health, and enhanced general well-being. In contrast, insecure, unstable, volatile relationships provide a profoundly negative impact by tending to increase stress and influencing both mental and physical illness.[7]

The people you gravitate toward magnetize to you for a reason, and you to them. However, even with this being true, you do have a choice in the matter. The unconscious driving forces that pull you toward certain relationships and away from others can be overridden by conscious awareness of your implicit relational patterning. Once you become aware of the distorted perception through which you perceive desirable relationships, you empower yourself to make different choices with stronger intentionality. Therapy is a great tool for helping you gain mindful awareness, and it will provide you with a plethora of resources to navigate relationships differently with your new perception intact.

Loneliness

Whether you find yourself in codependency, interdependency, or any other relational dynamic, it's safe to say that you probably pursue the connections you do in order to stave away the undesirable fear of loneliness that may be lurking somewhere in the deep corners of your psyche. Loneliness is not the same as solitude. *Solitude* is chosen aloneness that provides peace, reflection, and the spaciousness for Self-connection. Solitude is healthy and nourishing for your nervous system and your psyche on many levels. Theologian and philosopher Paul Tillich differentiates that solitude involves a positive experience of *being* alone, likely based on choice, while loneliness surfaces as the pain of *feeling* alone.[8]

The pain of loneliness is familiar to all humans, and most of us would rather not feel it. This is why we tend to strenuously work to avoid it. Loneliness is the heavy feeling of aloneness without choice. It is a cobwebbed emptiness where a person feels outside, excluded, and irrelevant. This is why so many people run toward commitment in an effort to stave off loneliness, sometimes getting cobbled up in dynamics like codependency before they understand how to construct truly healthy relationships. In addition to the downright awful emotional and psychological experience of loneliness, studies have shown it to be really detrimental for the physical body as well.

In her book *The Lonely Century*, Noreena Hertz documents several striking negative health outcomes of loneliness that may surprise you. She reports that loneliness is comparable to smoking fifteen cigarettes per day and is more hazardous to your health than obesity.[9] I don't know about you, but when I hear statistics like this it stops me in my tracks and inspires me to look twice at the quality of my relationships. Remember, too, that loneliness is not always the experience of *being* alone—it's *feeling* alone. Sometimes the loneliest times in a person's life happen when they are immersed in a crowd of people or seated at a family dinner table. Despite having warm bodies on all sides, they feel utterly unseen, unimportant, misunderstood, and undervalued. In this way, loneliness can be an individual perception rather than an objective reality agreed upon by others. No one can tell you if you feel lonely and with whom. That's for you to discern honestly for yourself and rectify.

> **How-To Tip**   Journal about loneliness and solitude and then create imagery. Notice when you have experienced each and with whom. Is there a moment when one tips into the other? Consider drawing yourself on one side of the page in a representation of loneliness. Perhaps you are alone or with someone you feel disconnected from. Your drawing may indicate feelings of emptiness and sadness (using the colors that represent these emotions). On the other side of the page, draw your depiction of solitude. Maybe you are still alone but this time drawn with colors that represent growth and happiness. In the center of the page, the "tipping point," explore what supports your transition from loneliness to solitude (such as self-love, creative expression, or escaping into a good book).

As long as you have your freedom, you have the ability to choose your relationships. You can cultivate more connections if you feel your social net is wearing thin, and pour extra love into your most meaningful connections to strengthen and fortify them. You have the power to move away from dynamics where you feel lonely. But what about individuals who no longer possess freedom, like convicts and prisoners? University of California Santa Cruz professor Craig Haney explored this question by studying the grave consequences of extreme loneliness that are instigated by prolonged solitary confinement among prison inmates. Sadly, Haney's research revealed that human beings who are left alone without connection, touch, or exposure to other people typically experience madness and behave in inhuman ways. Despite their crimes, some of which were abhorrent, Haney concluded that forced loneliness resulting from extended periods of solitary confinement is far too severe a consequence to serve as punishment for any human being—even the worst of criminals. The truth for all of our kind is that we deteriorate into unrecognizable creatures when we lack access to other human beings.[10] Because of this, loneliness should never be used as a consequence. It is painful enough to feel the stirrings of isolation so common in everyday life without exacerbating it with solitary confinement or any other extreme separation we may self-impose—even outside the walls of a federal prison.

Whether you are navigating loneliness, codependency, or any other relational dynamic, it is crucial to keep pivoting toward alignment in your connections for the sake of your own health and that of any others in your orbit. When you commit to healing your inner wounds and learning to healthfully relate to others, you can much more easily participate in strong, lasting relationships that benefit all involved. Even including the many flaws inherent in all interpersonal dynamics, relational commitment is a beautiful thing. Take it from me—I've been in a committed partnership with my husband for over years at this point, so you could say I'm a fan. I also feel deeply committed to my children and other family members, my closest friends, and my clients and colleagues who are dear to my heart. I'm also profoundly committed to my Self. With all that being said, I have shed my fair share of outdated commitments that drifted too far out of alignment to recover. Friendships, family relationships, belief systems, and even a thriving business fell by the wayside as I pivoted my commitments over the years. Yes, there was grief. I encountered doubts and uncertainty before arriving at clarity. I surfed many waves of confusion along the way. But every time I let go of a commitment that had grown stale, it served me well to have done so in the long run. Every single time.

When you consider commitment as a flexible quality that you can weave into your most meaningful relationships and life experiences like golden thread through a tapestry, you can see its abundant gifts. Even if the commitment is short lived, it will contribute to your life in ways that will eventually impact the whole of your being, regardless of its ambiguity in the moment. Whether we like it or not—whether we admit it or not—human beings tend to leave their marks on one another. If you maintain a growth perspective, you will see how the dynamics you have committed to over time helped to shape the person you have become—for better or worse. Commitment is like glue in both the best way possible and the worst. It can bond you to things and people who are important to you, and it can also keep you stuck where you no longer feel aligned. The trick is learning to discern which commitments are worth keeping and which would better serve you in hindsight. Remember, what worked yesterday or last year may or may not work today. Taking stock of which commitments to save and which to shed is a Now experience you must discern in the moment you are in. In the next chapter we'll discuss how to identify toxic relationships and healthfully end commitments with people who harm you.

CHAPTER 11

When Relationships Go South

It can be a slow, numb decline or a rapid snap of instantaneous rupture. Either way you know unquestionably when things go south in a relationship. Sometimes it takes a while for the mind, body, and heart to agree that something is wrong. In other situations, nothing has ever rung so true to the entirety of your being as the need to eradicate the problem at hand.

When a relationship starts turning sour, it is common for people to throw everything they've got at it in an effort to either save the relationship or distract themselves from the pain of its demise. Like anything else, there are healthy and unhealthy iterations of this. Healthy last-ditch efforts can sometimes look like:

- Initiating counseling, therapy, or coaching (individual, couples, and/or group)
- Lovingly confrontational conversations
- Creating space to connect for the purpose of identifying and working through problems together
- Joint creative expression like art making or journaling for reflection and insight
- Participating in a group retreat or another community-based support network

Less healthy endeavors, or in many cases radically unhealthy behaviors, used to stave off the discomfort of the relational downward spiral can include (but are not limited to):

- Numbing with substances or other behaviors that dull your awareness of the problem
- Trying to fix the problem by having a baby, buying a new home or car, or other such Band-Aid behaviors that neglect the root cause of the issue
- Projecting blame, aggression, manipulation, shame, guilt, or any other avoidant emotional response toward the other person
- Pretending that there is no problem and running away from the other person (physically or emotionally) when issues get triggered
- Gossiping (talking negatively about your counterpart to others) or triangulating (placing another person in the middle of the situation and avoiding direct communication)
- Refusing to do your inner work to discover how you might be playing into the interpersonal problems

If you use these unhealthy mechanisms (or any others I didn't mention) to cope with your dysfunctional relationship(s), it is important to nip them in the bud as soon as possible so they don't spiral into severe problems that impact your and/or others' health and safety. If you are unsure if you or a loved one is headed toward danger in their usage of maladaptive coping measures, I urge you to consider two questions that undeniably identify when there's a problem that requires extra help:

1) Does your substance use, avoidance of self-reflection, denial, or manipulative behavior interfere with your daily functioning? This means that you are unable to effectively care for yourself and your dependents, do a good job at work, reliably fulfill your responsibilities (like paying bills and filling your

refrigerator), and other basic elements of adult functioning.

2) Does your coping regularly make you feel shame, guilt, or regret? You could feel these emotions as a dull sensation throughout the day or acutely in specific moments of stress, tension, or even relaxation (like when you're trying to fall asleep).

If you answer "yes" to one or both of these questions, it might be time to bring in extra support because your coping skills could be escalating into a bigger problem. The discomfort of a painful relationship can easily plant seeds for managing your stress that unintentionally grow into deep mental health issues that require professional support. Therapy is a great way to explore the barriers you may have put in place to avoid the discomfort of a toxic or misaligned relationship. Be mindful to seek licensed therapists for situations like these—not coaches— because coaches lack the clinical skillset and professional regulation that a credentialed therapist will provide to support trauma healing, mental health struggles, and psychological issues. You can find local or remote individual, couples, and group therapy resources easily online or with a referral from your primary doctor. If a close friend has gone through something similar, their vote of confidence in a specific provider can also direct you toward a trusted professional. If your substance use is getting out of hand and starting to rule your life, consider initiating therapy with a certified addiction counselor (CAC), attending alcoholics anonymous (AA) meetings, or checking into a substance abuse treatment program if necessary. And always, if you are having thoughts of suicide please call the suicide and crisis hotline at 988, go to your nearest emergency room, or dial 911 for immediate help. As my middle-school gym teacher wired into my brain with her consistent mental health teaching when I was a pre-teen, *suicide is a permanent solution for a temporary problem*. There is always help available, and there are always options for you—no matter how dark life may seem.

Once you take ownership of the mechanisms you use to tolerate the discomfort of a failing relationship, you can more easily confront and heal them. If denial is your thing, you'll want to work toward acceptance. If you tend toward fear and overwhelm, calming your nervous system would be a priority. On the journey from uncertainty to clarity, you may discover that questions lead to more questions, and things can get harder before they get easier. That's okay. Relationships can be complex and messy when the conditioning and unhealed shadow material of those involved mesh together. Moving through a misaligned dynamic with the intention to regain health and balance (with or without the continuation of the relationship) is a layered process that requires patience and care.

When you feel grief, frustration, sadness, anger, or any other complex cocktail of emotions in response to a derailed relationship, it's easy to feel consumed by the experience. People often find themselves ruminating and obsessing, thinking of nothing else, and talking to anyone who will listen about the hardship of their relationship. In such situations, I encourage taking a *macro/micro* perspective to keep the scales balanced between each view. Here's what I mean:

When most of the globe was strictly locked down in quarantine during the spring of 2020 when the COVID-19 pandemic hit, I saw a video of Earth from the International Space Station (ISS). In stark contrast to the deep existential dread and fear that pulsed through my own body (and the bodies of many others around the world) in response to the mysterious virus that swept through our cities, our planet looked peaceful from space. Earth just floated on, a blue-green gem against the starry backdrop of the Milky Way galaxy. Zero-gravity astronauts couldn't see a trace of COVID-19 from the ISS. As I watched the video I thought, "Our problems are so insignificant compared to the vastness of space and everything in existence beyond our limited human awareness." It occurred to me that no matter how massive something feels in the moment, if you can't see it from the ISS, it really isn't as big of an issue as it seems to be in the greater story of the incomprehensibly vast universe. Thinking on this *macro* level helps me reorient myself with the problems I face (in relationships and elsewhere) here on Earth. It helps me re-member that I am a single drop in an endless ocean of time and space that existed long before I came along with my personal issues, and will continue long after I'm gone. Recognizing the *macro* helps me refrain from making everything that hurts feel massive. Ultimately, centralizing my problems as the dramatic demise of the world by catastrophizing the stress of daily life is unhelpful, so I need to reel it in.

Here's the thing, though: I can't permanently live in the *macro* or I become aloof, disconnected, and apathetic. After all, why should a human being care about anything at all if they are only a drop in a timeless ocean, insignificant from outer space? This is where acknowledging the *micro* comes in. For each of us, through our limited 3D perspective of human life, our reality is as real as we understand it to be. Because of this, our pain hurts. Our drama feels disruptive. Our orientation to rela-tionship troubles, our efforts to live with purpose, and our choices and behaviors along the way all matter significantly within the universe of the drop of water each of us is. It was Rumi who explained that we are each not a drop in the ocean but the entire ocean in a drop.[1] Holding a *micro* perspective of the daily happenings of our lives, caring about them, and in-

WHEN RELATIONSHIPS GO SOUTH 205

vesting in the continual navigation of human life is part of the package deal we've each got to contend with.

It is only with balance between *macro* and *micro* that we can successfully hold space for both the smallness and largeness of the challenges we face in our relationships and outside of them. When things go south in a meaningful dynamic, you've got a choice. You can swing to either extreme in how you consider the experience, or you can hold a *macro/micro* perspective and source wisdom from each perspective with equanimity. You can acknowledge that a connection feels stress-filled and troublesome while also remembering that in the greater scheme of things it won't matter all that much if the relationship floats or sinks—or even if you yourself float or sink (I know, it's dark. I went there). Your existence and that of your relationship both hang somewhere in the massive balance of the Milky Way galaxy, which floats in the gigantic soup of outer space that is unfathomable in its size and workings. It matters and it doesn't. It doesn't and it does.

Counterbalancing extremes and contrasting perspectives is valuable when you are faced with challenges that demand your focus and attention. It helps you make choices and traverse your human experience without being flooded by emotions that paralyze or distort your thinking (like fear). With this mindset intact, you can remain aware that you must make choices and steer your life. Sometimes finding the middle path helps clear the emotional charge from your system so you can meet the moment that is unfolding before you. Then there's not much left to do but put one foot in front of another and move forward as best you can.

The next time you feel flooded by fear, anxiety, anger, or anything else, I invite you to ask yourself if your current challenge matters from the ISS or not. Then place your hand over your heart, feel the beating life-force energy of your existence, and validate that your pain is real and important. After a breath or two, you'll find that you can proceed in one way or another—even if only with baby steps.

> **How-To Tip**   Draw, paint, or collage the view of your personal life—its richness, beauty, issues, and pain—from the ISS. You might represent yourself as a tiny speck on the earth, a magnified symbol like a hurricane or community celebration, or even invisible from the outer-space vantage point. Then create a close-up image of your personal world, including things and people that fill your life and bring joy, drama, and everything in between. After you complete both images, juxtapose them and write about the macro/micro perspectives of your personal life in your journal. You may discover that what you thought was important seems strangely less so after observing it from the ISS perspective. Also, maybe something that before seemed trivial now has a new sense of importance. Try to keep an open mind and hold space for whatever emerges.

When to Grit and When to Quit

Even if it's not obvious from the ISS, circumstances certainly present where important decisions need to be made—sometimes monumental ones like *should we stay together or break up?* Or *Should I keep grinding toward that big promotion even though my job drains my soul and is killing me slowly?* Annie Duke is a professional poker player who discovered that poker presents a wildly accurate depiction of humanity, social behavior, and our sometimes inconvenient need to make massive decisions without always having the necessary information to do so. Think about it: secret keeping, blatant inability to see each other's cards, and strategizing about how much to invest and when to fold are applicable in both poker and life. Duke[2] impeccably draws this striking parallel and proudly self-identifies as a quitter—which I admire. Like my *mend* or *move on* choice point, she explains that knowing when to quit is crucial, despite our conditioning to hang on to things, people, and experiences that ultimately do not serve us.

Grit is when a person persists through a challenging situation to pursue something worthwhile. Grit—an admirable personal quality—has acquired a glowy aura in our productivity-driven society that often diminishes the importance of rest and authenticity. Recklessly defaulting to the assumption that grit is appropriate for every situation and relationship, however, only reinforces that we should all be perpetually striving. This mindset explains why so many people are burned out, resentful, and deeply unhappy. If you inquire honestly within yourself, you will likely discover that you maintain such adherence toward things and people you have either outgrown or never truly aligned with from the beginning. Hey, you're human and a product of the society you've been marinating in since birth. It doesn't make you wrong or bad. It makes you acculturated to specific social values and systemic beliefs about the function and purpose of relationships.

Here's where *quit* comes in. I'll speak to this concept in the ballpark of relationship dynamics, but please remember that it also applies to professional endeavors, belief systems, and anything else you white-knuckle grip in strenuous attachment. If you operate under the assumption that you must endure the tumult of what is clearly a misaligned relationship, it is important to follow Adam Grant's lead and "think again."[3] By questioning what you think you know about the things (and people) you think you know, you open space to update your beliefs and perceptions, learn where you might be wrong, and expose yourself to new information that could radically alter your life and relationships. Let's be honest—most people think they know that quitting is a bad thing. They inaccurately think it should be avoided if at all possible. Truthfully, though, sometimes it's better to quit. As any quitter knows, letting go of a tough fight can improve health, foster freedom, and feel simply relieving. Why is it so hard, then? There are two primary reasons why we do mental-emotional gymnastics to justify and bargain ourselves into sticking it out:

- First, we hate to walk away from something we have invested a lot of time, energy, love, and work in. This is the *sunk cost fallacy*, which Richard Thaler[4] identifies as being when people become more attached to something after they have invested something of value (money, time, effort, etc.) into it.
- Second, we fear that we might later regret our decision to quit. Fearing regret can be a powerful motivator, but it can also keep you profoundly stuck.

Here's the deal: Nobody knows what lies ahead in the mysterious unlived future (crystal ball psychics exempt). The best we can do is source from the information at hand, built from past experiences and present wisdom gained from those experiences, and make choices we believe will serve our future good. If the thought of quitting has so much as peeked its unwelcome head over the horizon of your imagination, it's only fair to your future Self that you honestly consider why. Realistically, if you've never thought of quitting, you can likely discern that you are either happy in your present circumstances or in a deep, dark hole of denial that keeps you from Self-honesty. If you can be transparent with yourself and acknowledge fleeting thoughts about quitting, or if my broaching this topic has piqued your interest in association to a specific relationship, you've probably been tiptoeing around a significant issue for quite some time.

If you feel called out, good. This work is about applying authentic integrity to clearly identify relational misalignment in the service of correction. The tipping point between *grit* and *quit* might seem nuanced, but truthfully it's probably been a lengthy road of denial and avoidance that finally culminated at a breaking point where you feel ready to do the tough thing and walk away.

> **How-To Tip**   What rises to the surface as you read about grit/quit? Maybe a certain relationship keeps coming to mind that you have been struggling with. You might be thinking about the experience of a friend or loved one you observed going through this, or possibly you're thinking about a connection you have already ended. Journal about resistance, fear, or emotional charge surrounding both "grit" and "quit" and the tipping point where one becomes the other.

Endings

I often get caught up in thinking that things will last forever—large and small things alike. I fear that a splotchy skin rash will haunt me for the rest of my life. I hope that today's meaningful friendship will remain cherished and nutritive forever. I wonder if I will forever be an introvert who enjoys alone time more than 99 percent of the people I know. Forever, forever, forever. I am so wrong about all of these things. How could I believe that anything is forever when I have a lifetime of proof to the contrary? And yet . . .

I have learned to appreciate my forever-thinking as a form of self-protection. If there is something wonderful in my life, the fear of losing it—now or ever—feels terrifying. It protects me to bundle it in hope and attach *forever* to anything I'm frightened to lose. Conversely, if something scary is happening, my forever-thinking is a protective mechanism that prepares me, for my own good, to learn to live with the hardship long term (even if it disappears the very next day, to my relief and surprise).

Nothing is forever, even when you have a relationship you hope will endure that long. Endings happen. They are as natural to our life cycle as beginnings, and sacred within the ebb and flow of nature. That being said, endings can be painful, confusing, awkward, and a whole host of other things. Riddle me this: Why is it that we can be more or less accepting of the end of fifth grade, the end of a vacation, or the end of a book and absolutely defiant about the end of a relationship? I think it's the people thing. Once our hearts and minds mingle with those of others, complication sets in. We get attached. Human beings are social creatures. The missing piece for many, however, is the difference between love and attachment—and no, they are not the same thing. *Love* is an emotion. *Attachment* is a biological process used for safety. When a person gets attached—be it to a material item, an idea, or another person—they equate that attachment with security. Part of their psyche believes that the thing (or person) they attach to will keep them safe and out of serious trouble that could threaten their existence. I know it sounds dramatic, but that's the nervous system. It is wired for your survival and the continuation of our species, and it doesn't care one bit about how dramatic it seems.

When you get attached, for better or worse (inevitably, as Buddhist psychology teaches, it is always for the worse because attachment causes suffering), and that attachment must end, stress and devastation can be right around the corner. Losing something (or someone) you associate with your comfortable rhythms of safety and stability, something predictable and known, can feel scary and destabilizing. But that's not a good enough reason to remain attached when your health and growth require an ending.

The closure I have created for my misaligned relationships taught me valuable lessons about how I want to be treated, the types of people I am willing to grant access to me, and the participation I will and won't offer toward the lives of others. It is okay to be clear that you will allow in your life only love and connection that nourish and support, reciprocate and collaborate, offer kindness, and share compassion. As you release ties to those who are misaligned with these intentions, you open space for new relationships that can offer the connection your heart, body, and soul require. When you say a final goodbye, you free the other person to fulfill their needs for connection elsewhere, someplace more aligned with their values and priorities. If a fruitful bond from the past no longer exists, you can cut ties between yourself and anyone who holds you small. This can be done with love and gratitude for the past and hope for the potential allowed by saying goodbye. If your paths should cross down the line, you can greet each other with the kindness of old friends who once shared something meaningful. Practice seeing this process as a helpful lesson about the freedom you require and the degree of love you deserve.

Estrangement

There are many cultural messages that make estrangement, the cutting of ties with another (most often a family member), a topic of stress and controversy. Narratives like *blood is thicker than water* and *but you only have one (mother, father, sibling, whomever)* shame and invalidate a person's decision to step away from a relationship that feels irreparable and harmful to them.

When someone says, *But she's my mother! How could I cut off contact with my mother?* I respond by saying, *But you're her daughter! How could she place you in a position where you feel that cutting of contact is the choice you need to make?*

Estrangement is most common in families because familial relationships carry the strongest expectation for lifelong bonds. Regardless of the many sayings about how people should never walk away from family, closing the door (temporarily or permanently) is realistic for many people—especially those who have endured long-standing abuse and those who identify as cycle breakers.

There are two types of estrangement. The first is *emotional estrangement*, where a person disconnects emotionally from someone they deem unsafe or unhealthy for them. They may appear to go through the motions of connection, but their true inner Self is walled off and protected with barriers that resist emotional intimacy in the relationship. The second type of estrangement is *physical estrangement*, where a person goes no-contact with someone they wish to remove from their life either temporarily or permanently. No-contact relationships have no physical contact, phone calls, shared experiences, or emotional connection. The term *low-contact* defines an in-between scenario where participants maintain brief contact that remains emotionally guarded while they are mostly separated from one another's lives. If you have gone no-contact with someone, you likely understand that when a person arrives at the difficult decision to physically estrange from another (or a group), they have undoubtedly tried everything possible for years or decades to avoid making this final decision. Most often, physical estrangement is a last choice when someone feels that their health, safety, and/or stability will be significantly compromised if they remain in the relationship. It can feel like an ultimatum a person hoped to never have to face, where they must choose between their Self and the other person. It can feel so intense that I have heard clients explain it as being life or death.

Dr. Sherrie Campbell[5] draws a parallel between a person who has estranged from their family and a paraplegic person who no longer has use of their legs. Both scenarios are handicaps of differing kinds—one physical, one relational. Similar to the paraplegic person's legs in most cases, an estranged person's family members still exist—they just lack functionality in any meaningful way. Like legs that cannot communicate with the brain and nervous system due to the irreparable damage that caused the injury, cut-off family members can no longer maintain contact with the estranged person's most vital Self—even though the person still feels the weight of their existence. An estranged person remembers when they had full utilization of this capacity, like a paraplegic person may have memories of life before their injury, but this specific loss of functionality must be grieved as the person learns to live without it.

Tori's Story of Estrangement

Tori hardly knew what her favorite color was when I first met her, let alone her emotional boundaries. She had survived a lifetime of insidious manipulation and psycho-emotional abuse from her narcissistic mother, combined with the emotional immaturity of her deeply unhealed father who stood by the wayside and allowed Tori's abuse to persist without ever protecting her. Tori's younger brother remained compliant with her parents' dysfunction, so he became aligned with the distorted relationship dynamics that perpetuated the projection that Tori was the bad, wrong, difficult, troublesome problem child.

In her early thirties, Tori asked for my help managing her familial relationships. It is always a red flag for me when a client's intention is to *manage* or *deal with* difficult relationships. This insinuates to me that the person feels, on some level, that the relationships are not healthy connections between open-hearted people. Instead they likely know the dynamics to be dysfunctional, which ultimately brings the person to believe that they themselves must change in order to achieve peace within the system. Nedra Glover Tawwab explains[6] that you are not keeping the peace if the other person is the only one at peace and you are miserable. Much to the dismay of chronic people pleasers, one person's effort (no matter how extreme it may be) is insufficient to create a healthy relationship. Every interpersonal connection is a relational tango.

Back to Tori: We worked together for over ten years on the many layers of shame, insecurity, fear, guilt, and confusion that kept her trauma bonded to her unhealthy and abusive parents. Tori navigated difficult conversations, intentional boundary setting, grief when her boundaries and needs were continually disregarded, fearful experiences related to her parents' treatment of her children, and much more. Tori's psyche repeatedly sifted through evidence from every stage of her life, processed this information at intricate depths, and received confirmation from our sessions (as well as countless books, podcasts, and conversations with trusted loved ones) that her experiences were abusive and traumatic. Finally, she arrived at the immensely painful decision that she could no longer expose herself, her spouse, and her children to the dangerous toxicity of her parents and sibling. After realizing that she had unconsciously been in the process of emotional estrangement from her biological family for years, Tori chose to step into full-blown physical estrangement and go no-contact with her parents and brother.

This decision was not easy for Tori. It came after decades of pain and years of intentional healing and growth work that bolstered her advocacy for the safety of herself and the family she created with her spouse. It was a good thing Tori was certain about her decision and backed with the confidence she had acquired from her long inner work process. In vindictive rage, Tori's biological family reacted to her choice with psychological warfare. She dodged hate mail, love bombing, shame and blame, and aggressive manipulation of every color of the rainbow. Her parents recruited extended family members to advocate for Tori's self-abandonment, urging her to change her mind and return to the norm for the sake of the greater whole. Loved ones Tori had treasured in the past were weaponized against her by her mastermind manipulative mother, using hurtful tactics and inappropriate blame against Tori that nearly brought her to her knees on many occasions—but it didn't. Each time Tori confronted another toxic blow, her decision to estrange was confirmed and reinforced. Her parents' and brother's unhealthy responses to Tori's boundaries, without ever asking how they hurt her or contributed to her decision, affirmed that they were dangerous for her and her most cherished loved ones. Tori stayed the course. Although the arsenal of poisonous daggers sent by her family never completely ceased, Tori learned to shield herself from them effectively and live free from a system that would have undoubtedly drowned her in its toxicity.

Tori's story illustrates the complexity inherent in a decision to estrange and also demonstrates the necessity for such relationships to end for the sanity and health of the person in harm's way. Unfortunately, it's not enough to want strong relationships and work toward them on your own. You cannot create wholesome dynamics with people who are unwilling to behave healthily because they are so unhealed, defensive, aggressive, abusive, and shrouded in denial. Certain relationships end in estrangement because it is the only way for a person to move forward in one piece, with their dignity intact, and without stress-induced cancer, mental health disorders, or hypertension derived from longtime exposure to toxic people.

Ella's Story

Another client of mine, Ella, was absolutely baffled at the disparity time and experience had created in the way she felt about her mother. For many years she had explored and healed the negative impact on her psyche and emotional body from years of abuse in this primary relationship. In hindsight, Ella could see the unfoldment of her wounding and subsequent inner repair with a particular grace I am still in admiration of.

Ella reached a breaking point in her early forties where estrangement from her mother felt like the only healthy option left for her. In one of our sessions she shared a memory of when she was a little girl, maybe eight or ten. Ella secretly left her mother heartfelt love notes on her pillow. She explained that she felt such love for her mother at that time and fear that she would ever lose her, and she just had to express it. She then went on to share that as an adult, looking back at the years of trauma and abuse, Ella realized her mother never so much as acknowledged her love notes when she was a girl, let alone reciprocated them.

As Ella integrated the memory of her mother's lack of response toward her outpouring of love, she clearly perceived the negative impacts she had been forced to tolerate in her early relationship with her primary caregiver. Often, children (and adults, too) give the kind of love to others they deeply wish to receive themselves. By writing love notes to her mother and leaving them in a place where she imagined her mother would be surprised and delighted to discover them, Ella attempted to show her mother the kind of love that would feel good for Ella herself to receive. Imagine the joy a little girl might feel upon approaching her bed at the end of the day to find a sweet note written by her mother. This was Ella's fantasy and yearning, even if she did not cognitively understand it at the time. By not receiving recognition, appreciation, or reciprocity in the expression of her love, Ella developed a core wound related to her worth and the untrustworthy nature of relationships that required years of therapy in adulthood to identify and heal.

The Right to Choose

When I speak with people who are navigating estrangement, I often remind them that as adults they have the right to choose whom they allow in their lives. Nobody, regardless of their familial standing, is entitled to your time, love, body, or energy. Full stop. It is a privilege to be in your life. If anyone makes you feel otherwise, that is a relationship worth looking at. People who consider estrangement often confuse themselves with a thorough questioning process that can last for years. They want to know that they tried everything possible and made the only healthy decision available before choosing to go no-contact. It is okay for this process to have many layers that take time and professional support to sift through, like in Tori's case. You have to be truly ready when you commit to no-contact status, especially if you have children who will be impacted by your decision. If you wonder what would make a person estrange from another, here are several common reasons:

- When a person has endured abuse of any kind (physical, mental, psychological, sexual, spiritual) and they are no longer willing tolerate maltreatment.
- When they have tried everything imaginable to heal the relationship, but the other person is unwilling or unable to put forth effort to do the same.
- A family's blatant, continuous criticism, judgment, or negativity toward the chosen spouse or partner of their adult child.
- A clash of values so extreme that there is no longer common ground for connection without igniting severe arguments, disagreements, or conflict.
- Exhaustion and depletion when a person has used every tool and resource accessible to them without seeing healthy change in the relationship, and the effort has rendered them empty.
- The last straw has crumbled, and nothing remains to connect people who have been through extensive drama and trauma together to the point where it feels impossible to continue trying.
- A person has changed and grown to such an extent that their healthy lifestyle and behaviors are unrecognizable to their unhealthy family, so they get scapegoated and rejected.

If you are at the end of your rope with a family member or close relationship and you are considering estrangement, please know that you are not alone. It can be a scary time in a person's life when they end a relationship with the complex underpinnings of family origins or lifelong bonding. Seek as much help, resourcing, healthy connection, therapeutic support, and skill building as possible to fortify and sustain you on this journey. From my heart to yours, I hope you'll remember these truths:

- You deserve to be treated with kindness and respect from every relationship in your life—no exceptions.
- Keep moving forward toward people and experiences that bring out the light in you.
- Freedom and peace are possible for you.
- Never give up on yourself. Keep choosing You.
- Protecting your children from the people who hurt you is a healthy choice.
- It is not your responsibility to manage other people's reactions to your decisions.
- If you feel doubtful, confused, or insecure about your choice, remind yourself of how you came to the decision to estrange. Ask the loved ones who have supported you throughout your journey to remind you of your drive toward health and safety.

How-To Tip It is common to feel doubt and insecurity when navigating estrangement. Many who go no-contact experience fear because estrangement feels final and irreversible. Because of this, it can help to revisit evidence that led you to your decision. Write a list of every memory and experience you have of pain in the relationship you are ending. Go back as far as possible and create a complete list that fully captures all you have been through. When you read your list in moments of doubt or fear, you will remember why you have chosen this path.

Here's a visual metaphor that helps with understanding the cyclical nature of relational beginnings and endings. Imagine that life presents as a path, like a yellow brick road for you to traverse. All that surrounds the path represents your relationships and experiences. At the very beginning of the yellow brick road, you are given a small bouquet of flowers that are intended to offer you comfort, pleasure, and something to occupy your hands for a while. This bouquet represents the grouping of your earliest caregivers and connections (a rose for Mom, a daisy for Dad, a lilac for Grandma . . . you get the point). Along the way, you might notice other flowers you like, and you may choose to add them to your bundle (a lily for a new friend, a sunflower for your first-grade teacher, etc.). When you insert fresh stems, you might see that certain blossoms have wilted or died, so you may choose to remove those and leave them behind as you venture forward. This represents relationships that have served their purpose or expired. Some flowers might nestle in for the long walk, and others may fall to the ground after only a brief time in the bouquet.

Some of the relationship-flowers you were born with, while others you pluck and integrate along your travels. Each flower (i.e., relationship) serves a purpose along the road of your life for however long you choose to carry it. If you collect more flowers than you can carry, you might decide to thread stems through your hair or bundle them in your pockets, but eventually you will run out of room. If you refuse to set aside the blossoms that have died along the way, you will be carrying armfuls of wilted blooms that bring only the memory of what once was without contributing further vitality to your life. You may choose to carry a limited number of flowers so that your arms can be free to swing in the breeze, or you may choose to stuff yourself so full of bouquets (social interactions) that you can hardly see the path ahead. You may choose to carry only stems without thorns to protect yourself from the prickles that adorn blossoms too beautiful to exist without soldiers, or you might learn to respectfully hold the thorns so as not to sacrifice the beauty you seek. If you're still hanging with me through this rabbit hole metaphor, say "I."

The point of my musings about flowers, thorns, and yellow brick roads is meant to teach you that it's okay to pick up new relationships as you venture forward in your life. It is also acceptable to gently release those who no longer serve your highest good. Although it can be painful to end long-standing relationships that were built from your effort, time, energy, and love, *forever* is not a requirement for relationships—nor is it realistic for many connections.

How-To Tip   Draw yourself with your current relationships represented by a flower bouquet in your hands. Represent each relationship as a flower, weed, or decorative branch of leaves. Consider metaphorical qualities when deciding if each relationship is delicate/resilient, bold/soft, prickly/gentle, large/small, etc. Bring thoughtful attention to how you draw yourself. Are you walking with ease or struggle? Is your face smiling or stressed? Are your arms tired from carrying too many flowers or grazing the grass for new stems to pluck? Journal about your finished product and creative process for deeper insight.

CHAPTER 12

When It's More Than the Two of You

When each of my children was born, I opened an email account for them—and not just to snag theirname@gmail.com for their future use. Throughout the years, it has been my intention to use these accounts to write notes to the future Selves of my children—notes they will be granted access to when they seem old enough and ready for them. At first, I sent emails with baby pictures accompanied by oohs and aws of their adorableness and how sweet it is to be their mom. Over time, as life has unfolded both for me as their mother and for them as budding personalities emerging into their agency and sovereignty, the accounts have become places where I write to my kids about more serious matters. I choose to impart teachings from my own experiences, life lessons I pick up along the way, and even explanations that detail my thinking when I make important decisions that impact their lives.

As I write this book my children are nine and eleven, and I still write emails to their future Selves. I don't write to their rosy-cheeked chubby-wrist child Selves—I write to the adults they will become. I imagine my children growing into their own, developing their Self-concepts and worldviews based on their life experiences. Sure, it is my job as their mother to melt over their adorableness and gush about how proud I am of their ski team trophies and first days of school. Also, it is my responsibility to teach my kids the tricky stuff—the nuanced, subtle, complicated, sometimes heartbreaking reality of what it means to be a human in this often inconceivably complex world we share. Among other lessons, I choose to teach my children how to spot relationship toxicity and sidestep or extricate from it. I want them to know what to do when grief strikes, crisis explodes, or love pulls them down so strongly that they feel tempted to never resurface. I view my emails as a form of modeling where I communicate with my dear ones about the values of my heart. Modeling is an important facet of parenting because your children are always watching you, listening to you, observing how you move through the world, and building their own narratives from the life you live before their eyes. In other words, whether you realize it or not, whether you intend to or not, as a parent you are constantly teaching by example in large and small ways (no pressure, winky smiley face).

I take this responsibility seriously. I have come to understand that setting an example for my children (modeling) includes three important aspects:

1. **Consciousness:** I must live my life in a way I can be proud of so that my children observe the real-time actions, behaviors, beliefs, practices, and values of an adult they trust.

2. **Continuity:** I must reinforce my actions, words, behaviors, and values with explanations for why I choose them in conversation with my children at the level they are developmentally ready for. This means that I must repeat the same conversations with my kids, but at different levels of intensity, vulnerability, and detail as they grow, mature, and likely ask more complex questions.

3. **Trust:** I must trust that I modeled my parental teachings to the best of my ability and that I have solidly committed to continue living in a way I can be proud of. With this knowledge intact, I will allow my children to claim their agency and autonomy as they feel ready to do so, and I will allow them the freedom to make their own decisions when they are developmentally prepared.

It is my hope that when I hand over the passwords to their email accounts, my children will interpret my messages as guideposts based on the learnings I have acquired, and hopefully my words will provide a little clarity. Possibly my kids will learn from my mistakes, benefit from my glimmers of wisdom, and gain new threads of understanding about where they came from. Maybe, if the stars align, my emails might alleviate some suffering for my children. And isn't that the end goal anyway? To shape the minds and hearts of healthy kids who then go on to evolve the human species by doing things differently (and better) than those who came before them. For me, that's the goal.

If you are a parent (or a nonparental primary caregiver), you likely feel the intense gaze of your children upon you. You may even sense the impact your choices have on them. Your decisions about your career, substance use, material wealth, and relationships are all relevant to your youngsters. Perhaps your children are still so little that they seem light-years away from comprehending your life decisions. Regardless of their age or developmental readiness, remember that your children are filing away what they witness and learn from you (even subconsciously) as they build their worldview and discern their place in the grand order of things.

In the realm of relationships, it is no secret that your inter-personal conflicts, ruptures, breakups, and estrangements affect the myriad of people in your life—especially those with a front-row seat to the relationship in discussion (be they your children, members of your friend group, your employees, or others). If you do not have children, you can bet that there are other loved ones who feel the effects, positive or negative, of your relational dysfunction. Can you pinpoint who these people may be?

> **How-To Tip**   Journal about people who are close enough to you to feel the impact of your relational distress. Note how awareness ripples out to these individuals or groups and how they experience your interpersonal discord. Make art about what it looks like for the ripples of your toxic and misaligned relationships to reach your loved ones. Perhaps they tint your connection with your children or friends in a darker hue. The ripples might consume other people in dust, water, or haze. Consider metaphorical qualities of elemental representations: Water could drown, fire could scathe, and smoke or dust could make it hard to breathe and see.

A very common form of third-party awareness of relational discord is the children of two parents who are in a dysfunctional (or even disintegrating) relationship. These are the little ones whose parents exist in a state of persistent drama, abuse, conflict, or divorce. With intimate exposure to their parents' relational conflict, due to close proximity and emotional ties, kids undoubtedly feel the negative ripples that emanate off parents who are profoundly unhappy together.

So what's a miserable parent to do when divorce seems like the best course of action? First of all, we must all accept that divorce is a reality in our modern world. Relationship conflict and disharmony are pervasive to the point where there is a certain normalcy to a child being exposed to arguing adults. How, then, can a parent best protect their children from the harmful effects of their own unhealed wounds that get triggered and re-wounded by their partner? Here are some ideas:

- Remember *modeling*? Your kids are always watching and listening, so you have a powerful opportunity to model how to have healthy conflict, how to seek outside help to support a relationship, which kinds of treatment are acceptable to tolerate and which are not, and when to leave an unhealthy connection.
- *Stick to your decisions*: Children are easily confused by parents who vacillate in their decisions and choices. This is because the majority of a child's life is based on the decision-making of their parents. A child can feel exceedingly unsafe and powerless when their parents are erratic in their decision-making process. This doesn't mean you have to be perfect and can never change your mind. Just try, to the best of your ability, to not communicate a final decision (especially if it is life-altering like a divorce or family estrangement) unless you can commit to sticking to the decision. Then deliver the information to your child honestly and with sensitivity. Allow them to ask questions and feel feelings about what you communicated and its subsequent impact on their new reality.
- *Resource for your child*: Sometimes, despite your best intentions, your child can get caught in the cross fire or have strong psychological or emotional responses to your decisions. This is when it is important to build a reliable resource toolkit for

your child by gathering the specific kinds of support that will benefit their mental, emotional, physical, and spiritual health. Maybe it's art therapy, play therapy, or talk therapy. Perhaps your child needs more unstructured time on weekends where they can be alone with their thoughts and play independently. Maybe your little one will benefit from a regular Sunday night dinner with their grandparents to help them feel connected to their wider family network. You may find that increasing your child's exposure to a spiritual or religious community might help them—or removal from such a community might be necessary if it feels misaligned. Choose two or three things to try, and focus on adorning your child with love and support to help them through the difficult time. It's okay to fail and flail while you experiment with what works best. It may take time and experimentation, and you certainly don't have to get it right the first time around. Just keep trying until you discover what brings your child the flavor of support they need.

- *Make yourself available*: Lean in when your child expresses discomfort related to uncertainty, change, sadness, or other emotional experiences. Be available to answer their questions honestly, spend extra time together doing things your child enjoys, and demonstrate that you are present and paying attention to their need for support and connection. No matter what happens in any of our lives, we all do a lot better when we feel connected to trusting, safe people. For your child, that's probably you.

My Children's Parent vs. My Parent's Child

Speaking of children and parents, there are two very different Selves that exist within me: the Me I am as my parents' child and the Me I am as my children's parent. Can you relate? In some ways there seems to be a gaping chasm between these two Selves and in others only a hairline fracture. Truthfully, these two versions of Me were built upon one another in a nonlinear fashion that moves backward and forward through time. Allow me to explain further.

Certain spiritual traditions based on reincarnation believe that babies choose their parents as teachers who will impart lessons their soul is ready to learn in the lifetime they incarnate in. Whether or not this belief system resonates for you, let's assume for now that we do not consciously choose the parents we are born to. I did not have the conscious choice to be born to my parents, even if subconsciously or spiritually I may have had a different agenda. It just seemed to happen, and *poof*, family. In contrast, I did consciously choose to become a mother. Circumstances certainly exist where a person becomes a parent accidentally or through traumatic sexual abuse leading to unwanted pregnancy, and I make no assumptions about the experiences (spiritual or otherwise) of people in such complex situations. For the purpose of this section, I speak to the experience of becoming a parent by means of either conscious choice and planning or spontaneous choice followed by actively embracing an unexpected pregnancy.

Returning to my choice to become a mother, herein lies the first difference between my Self as a child and my Self as a parent. Both relational dynamics serve as spiritual teachers of the highest order, revealing lessons both large and small and reflecting parts of myself back to me for growth and development.

Both my parents and my children have, hands down, been my most profound teachers—sometimes uncomfortably so. As my parents' child, however, I am notably smaller (psycho-emotionally) than in my experience of being my children's parent. Nature developed the parent-child linear structure to ensure successful evolution and continuation of our species by placing small, impressionable youngsters in the position to be groomed, taught, and prepared for life by the older and (hopefully) wiser generation. Sometimes transgenerational teaching works out the way nature intended—good parents raise well-adjusted children, and those children grow into healthy parents who nurture their own radiant children. Other times, trauma and relational discord distort the lessons a child receives from their parents. This isn't necessarily what nature intended, but it's reality. Sometimes bad stuff happens within a family. Because the power and dominance inherent in a parent-child dynamic is asymmetrical, parents inherently hold more control, influence, and authority than their child. This is crucial to consider when addressing relational family trauma across generations.

> **How-To Tip**   Journal about yourself as your parents' child and yourself as your children's parent. What similarities and differences do you notice? You may also wish to create a visual image that symbolizes the different positions of power within your family line. Consider drawing certain people larger, smaller, brighter, dimmer, more substantial, or less so in relationship to one another. Then simply spend time looking at your image and notice how the differing sizes, shapes, and expressions of power in your image land with you. Jot down the emotions that arise and consider bringing this image to a therapy session for further processing.

Right Relationship

A mentor of mine refers to the dynamic of largeness and small-ness as *right relationship* within a lineage where elders who came first hold a decisively larger energetic embodiment than those who come after. This allows prior generations to provide pro-tection and teaching while participating in nature's special de-sign to usher young ones through vulnerable childhood and into adulthood where they can hold bigness in relationship with their own descendants. When children learn life lessons (healthy or not) from their parents—consciously, unconsciously, or en-ergetically—it is as though the messages are wrapped around them in a bubble that is not of their making. Children are the receivers of the complex gifts of their educational legacy that can be healthy, toxic, and everything in between. From inside this bubble they learn what it means to be a human being on planet Earth. The bubble cocoons and marinates them in the energetics of their lineage without their explicit consent or awareness.

Years later, having developed into adults, grown children ful-fill the same role for their offspring. A bubble of their design encompasses their own children's physical, emotional, psycho-logical, and energetic fields. In this case, the once-child becomes the sender of wisdom with their offspring as the innocent receiver.

Throughout the generations, there is a certain order and se-quence by which energy must flow within a lineage to create resonant intergenerational rightness in an ancestral chain. This linear order is essential for each familial relationship to be in proper alignment within the lineage as a whole. *Right relation-ship* encompasses more than a parent, their child, and their child's child. It includes at least seven generations backward and forward from any one person through space and time. Visualize a line of people standing single file with the youngest generation first. Behind them stand their parents, behind those individuals stand their parents, and back and back through time. Like a multitiered flowing fountain, each generation pours down into the next, giving the subsequent generation information from the elders and offering an opportunity to integrate, embrace, or change what passes through to their own descendants. This flow is how a lineage is made. It can resemble a healthy fountain only if the relationships flow in the linear fashion of right relationship.

How-To Tip Are you living in right relationship within your lineage? Create a drawing that demonstrates the linear or nonlinear order of at least three generations in your lineage. Then process your image in writing, with your therapist, or with a trusted loved one.

Problems arise when kinks happen in a lineage, such as one generation trying to skip another, a younger descendant aiming for power over an elder, or a loss of integrity in the flow from one generation to another. In the grand order of things, no matter how old a child grows in adulthood, they will always be the child of their parent. No matter how much a child wants to supersede their parent, they must remember that they are that person's child. Of course there is wiggle room within this model that allows for different generations to care for and protect one another. There is also potential for a person to confront and challenge relatives outside of their own generation. Overall, though, a person must structurally understand that to maintain right relationship, a parent will always be a parent in the parent-child relationship. Additionally, the sequence of right relationship moves backward and forward further than just between parents and their children. For example, it is not right relationship for a grandparent to control the flow of energy between their adult child and their grandchild. This intergenerational interference will negatively imbalance a lineage. Grandparents must respect their adult children as the gatekeepers of their grandchildren. Conversely, children must remember the sanctity of their parents' role in the genetic line, regardless of the troubles that may arise relationally. Even if an adult child chooses to confront issues with their parents or estrange from them, they must continue to honor their parents with gratitude for bringing them into the world. Respect can still exist in situations of estrangement that honor right relationship, even if the relationship is not healthy enough to sustain. A person can remain grateful to their parents for giving them life while also choosing to discontinue the harmful relationship.

One example of a lineage that was painfully derailed from right relationship is the story of my client Victoria. After years of immense struggle and misalignment, Victoria no longer wished to tolerate repeated emotional abuse from her father, Eduardo. Eduardo had been cruel and manipulative throughout Victoria's life, and he projected harsh negativity toward Victoria's chosen partner for the entirety of their marriage. Victoria and her partner had two children together, whom they worried would be emotionally unsafe with Eduardo if they remained vulnerable to his toxic behavior or became the objects of his distorted fixation. Over time, Victoria tried everything she could think of to heal the ruptures and misunderstandings between herself and her father, but nothing worked. She finally acknowledged that she saw no way to keep herself and her family safe besides estranging from her father. Although Eduardo seemed content to let his daughter go, he was not accepting of being estranged from his grandchildren. Victoria noticed that the less energy Eduardo targeted toward her, the more he diverted his focus around her and attempted to contact his grandchildren without the consent of Victoria and her partner. Eduardo sent love letters to his grandchildren by postal mail and gooey texts to their devices. Victoria received a few letters from her father that she aptly called "hate mail" because they exuded only blame, shame, and accusation. She never received anything that expressed Eduardo's desire to heal their relationship, take accountability for harm he caused, or communicate about his desire to stay connected with Victoria's children. Eduardo simply sidetracked his stream of energy around his daughter and pummeled his grandchildren with love bombing—a manipulative behavior where narcissistic people (or others in dysfunctional relationships) shower someone with compliments, attention, and love-like expressions for the purpose of gaining control and power over them.

In Victoria's case, her father's circumnavigation of right relationship within the lineage and subsequent love bombing of his grandchildren created an intergenerational toxicity that was deeply disrespectful of Victoria's efforts to keep herself and her family safe. It was also profoundly dishonoring of Victoria as the mother of two innocent children who were being targeted like prey by their emotionally unwell grandfather. Eduardo's actions, in his anxiety and destabilization, resulted from his inability to healthfully navigate the ruptures between himself and his daughter. In his denial and avoidance of the severe dysfunction between himself and his daughter, Eduardo created a family dynamic where right relationship was both disregarded and demolished.

Had Eduardo maintained the emotional maturity to remain in right relationship within the lineage, he would have directly contacted his daughter to discuss the situation at hand and its possible solutions. Even if Victoria and Eduardo decided to end their father-daughter relationship, healthy access between Eduardo and his grandchildren may have been granted if he demonstrated the decency and respect to remain in right relationship with his daughter regarding the energetics at play. Through a great deal of therapeutic work, Victoria could eventually honor her father as one of her sacred biological parents. She remained grateful for the gift of life Eduardo gave her without feeling the need to maintain contact with him.

Victoria's story is a sad one, and an extreme case that is more common than you might imagine. Her experience illustrates the importance of intergenerational dignity within a family system—even when unrest develops in individual relationships. It turns out, as evidenced by Victoria's story and countless others, that there is a right way to handle conflict within an ancestral line. It's all about directness and flow from one generation to another without skipping any in between.

Situations that are out of sync with right relationship can initiate an avalanche of cascading emotional burdens within a lineage, such as in Victoria's case. They can also present in monetary and materialistic manifestations such as a case when a grandparent skips over their child in their estate plan and wills money to their grandchildren instead. This can also happen with precious legacy items such as jewelry, real estate, businesses, and other estate items as they get passed down through generations.

An example of a family that was out of right relationship between siblings is the story of James and Petra. After their parents' passing, the multimillion-dollar real estate empire from the prior generation was passed down to the siblings, but not equally. Petra was placed in a position of power by her father, who had been the sole decision-maker of the estate. In his will, the father named James as an equal partner when it came to the financial dividends and shares of the business, but he snuffed out his voice and power by making James a silent partner. Petra was given full decision-making power over the entire business regardless of what her brother thought or felt about her choices. By placing one sibling in power over the other, James and Petra's father jolted their lineage out of right relationship. As a natural consequence of the misalignment within the family, deep hurt, dysfunction, and resentment built within James that ultimately devastated the family with legal battles, irreparable estrangements, and the disintegration of the family business.

Balance and harmony are crucial in all of nature, and are present within the dynamics of human relationships and collective family energetics. When a lineage gets thrown out of balance in a disregard for right relationship, massive damage can be long-lasting and develop unforgivable wounds smack-dab in the center of a family's energetic bond. To avoid such disastrous outcomes, remember to maintain balance within families by making fairness, direct communication, and respectful consideration between generations a paramount consideration.

When intergenerational discord and patterns are at play, there is an exciting component that brings choice and intention into the mix: Although we lack choice about what teachings and energetic material we receive from our parents in our early years, many people awaken to their personal agency and reclaim their power to accept or deny access of those lineage patterns in adulthood. Even with autonomy in adulthood, the early messages, values, and beliefs we receive from our parents get embedded within us like elaborately woven threads in the tapestry of our psyches. This is where the transformative work of inner exploration and self-discovery offers each generation the potential to break free from unhealthy material from those prior.

You can become conscious about the specific energetics you wish to teach your children about the magical and dangerous world they have been born into, even if your lessons deviate greatly from the teachings of those before you. When you selectively choose which of your parents' teachings are valid, which are corrupt, which make sense, and which don't, you can sprinkle the lessons from prior generations amid your own teachings about life to your offspring.

> **How-To Tip**   Consider the freedom you have to do things differently from those who came before you. What will you do with that power? Journal about what qualities, beliefs, teachings, values, and priorities you will keep from prior generations, and which you will dispose of.

Ancestors, Descendants, and Epigenetics

Visualize a long silver chain that stretches across the length of a football field with one neon green link somewhere at its center. That neon link is you. You exist somewhere in the middle of a long line of ancestors who came before you and potential descendants who may come after you. Even if you do not procreate, it is highly likely that someone from your lineage will—a sibling, cousin, etc. This means that your lineage will most likely continue forward, even without your efforts (except in the case of an apocalypse or mass extinction of humanity, and let's hope neither of those happen any time soon). In addition to your long chain of links, imagine that the green grass of the football field is buried beneath billions of other chains just like yours. These are the lineages of everyone you know, as well as everyone you don't know and may never meet. When you choose to connect with someone, especially in an intimate relationship, you consciously or unconsciously contribute the material from your lineage chain in combination with theirs. That's a lot of behaviors, beliefs, practices, and issues—*baggage*—you each bring to the table of your shared experience that span so far back in time your brain can't fully grasp the magnitude.

How do we know this? The science of epigenetics teaches about the way different genes (passed down from generation to generation) express themselves within a person by turning on or off in response to various environmental factors. It is possible that you have a gene for Alzheimer's disease, though it may never express (turn on) if you maintain the healthy diet, low stress, and avoidance of other risk factors that activate the genetic expression of that particular portion of your DNA. It is now common knowledge that you pass genetic material to your descendants and can track heritable traits between generations. The granularity of how specific these genetic legacies are, and your power to intentionally redirect them, is the gift of epigenetics.

When your grandmother was five months pregnant with your mother, the genetic material that would eventually become you was present in your mother's fetal ovaries as one of her many eggs.[1] If your grandmother drank heavily or was exposed to environmental toxins during her pregnancy with your mother, those pollutants would trickle down to you in trace amounts. If your grandmother was buried under the heavy emotional bricks of depression, that genetic material (including the stress and emotional suffering it caused your grandmother) would pass to you. These examples show how your individual link connects to a long chain where genetic information, behaviors, emotions, and life experiences are more pervasively shared intergenerationally than science previously understood.

Before you start feeling anxious, upset, or even victimized by the ancestral hardships that trickled down to you, understand that you have the power to break patterns and heal ancestral suffering that predates you. This is where intentional inner work related to accountably, self-awareness, and transformative personal healing come into play—the work of becoming a *cycle breaker*. For a full master class on self-healing and cycle breaking, read my book *The Radiant Life Project: Awaken Your Purpose, Heal Your Past, and Transform Your Future*. To close this section, I'll leave you with a potent quote from Bruce Springsteen: "At the end of the day, the way we honor our parents and their efforts is by carrying on their blessings and doing our best not to pass forward their troubles. . . . Our children's sins should be their own. . . . We all have to learn and earn our own adulthood."[2] Now, if that's not the right relationship, I don't know what is.

> **How-To Tip**   Journal about how you have learned and earned your own adulthood. How are you passing forward the material of prior generations?
>
> **BONUS How-To Tip**   Create a drawing or painting that depicts your lineage among other ancestral lines on a giant football field, represented as long chains with many links. Then identify your unique link and color it brightly.

CHAPTER 13

The Six Relationship Tools You Won't Want to Leave Home Without

It's no secret that relationships can get derailed and suffer profound consequences when they are packed with trauma, projection, judgment, and carelessness. But that can't be all relationships, right? Close your eyes and visualize which of your relationships are working well. Think back to connections that went profoundly *right*, even if they may not have lasted for the long haul. I'm sure you can piece together your own conception of ideas about what fuels healthy, lasting connections that nourish and sustain you. In this chapter I will discuss my six personal favorites. Keep in mind that there are endless helpful qualities that nurture and grow healthy interpersonal bonds; this list is simply a starting place. You might discover that you need all six of these elements to foster the connection you require for your emotional health and safety, or feel free to pick and choose what aligns and leave what doesn't. You will likely notice that different bonds require more or less of each tool depending on their intimacy and intensity. Make this fit for you, for each of your relationships, with the understanding that every bond is different. Also, feel free to add any other essential ingredients you deem necessary for cultivating thriving dynamics in all of your diverse and important connections.

Tool #1: Communication

Right out of the gate I'll begin with a biggie—communication—because, let's be honest, if you don't effectively communicate there's just too much room for misunderstanding to take root and bloom into a massive disaster. When you feel misunderstood, it's nearly impossible for a relationship to be authentically safe regardless of whether it exists in the bedroom, at Thanksgiving dinner, at the office, or at your friend's bachelorette party. Not all communication is verbal, though in our highly cerebral society effective communication by means of thoughtfully chosen words is an important skillset to develop. In addition to infusing your words with clarity, consistency, kindness, and honesty, you must also consider what your nonverbal cues communicate to others (or don't communicate, in many cases). Nonverbal communication includes body language, insinuations, assumptions, behaviors, or actions that convey meaning without words. What is your eye contact (or lack thereof) saying? How about your body language? Notice if you tend to cross your arms or lean toward or away from someone during conversation. Notice where inaction has become a form of communication. How do you respond to bids for connection like casual touch, an inquiring smile, or the transmission of a humorous GIF? Your lack of action is a choice, and it sends as potent a message as paragraphs of words.

In addition to body language, it is also impactful to nonverbally communicate through energetic and emotional expression. I'll bet you can remember a time when you were in someone's presence and, although they may not have said anything rude or snarky, you felt a definite standoffish vibe or perceived criticism in their tone or energy. The subtle sciences study how we exude emotional and energetic material through our pores and in the frequencies surrounding our bodies. Even as modern science struggles to remain open to the possibility that consciousness extends beyond the physical body, most people would agree that they can sense when someone dislikes them, just as they can sense when someone is attracted to them, annoyed by them, or uncomfortable in their presence. All people constantly send and receive messages to connect, collaborate, discern threats and dangers, and navigate the complex interpersonal web within which we all belong. Remember, we were not given fangs or furry coats to survive—we were given each other. And communication, in all its shapes and forms, helps us develop the clarity and expression necessary to understand which relationships serve us and which we would be better off without.

When discussing communication, it is easy to fall into the trap of assuming that the signs and words you send out encapsulate your entire responsibility in this realm, but you would be mistaken. In my opinion, what you hear and receive from others is just as important as what you deliver. And, as it turns out, not all listening is equal. In her work on communication, Faye Doell teaches about the crucial difference between *listening to understand* and *listening to respond*. Certain types of listening function to provide an opening for someone to speak about themselves and their reflections (listening to respond). Alternately, listening with the intention to comprehend the interpersonal bigger picture, inclusive of nuance and varying perspectives between people, encompasses a deeper intention to perceive the situation (and everyone in it) with awareness and integration (listening to understand). Perhaps unsurprisingly, Doell's research[1] discovered that *listening to understand* tends to result in higher relationship satisfaction across-the-board than *listening to respond*. When you think about it, this makes perfect sense.

It's annoying to converse with someone who is listening only to the extent where they gain an opening to talk about themselves. This self-unaware, nonreciprocal way of interacting tends to result in relationship endings far more often than it contributes to satisfying connections that last. On the flip side, dynamics that prioritize intentional give-and-take of communication, with both parties sharing and receiving, are highly likely to make all people involved feel seen, heard, and cared for. When you listen with the desire to truly understand another person, your shared circumstances with them, and yourself as part of the puzzle, you gain a holistic comprehension of the relational happenings that allows for healthy troubleshooting and repair when dynamics get out of whack. If you only listen to respond, deeper understanding of the other person's feelings and experiences get lost beneath your agenda to only be heard. This primes a dynamic for abrasive escalation rather than connection based on compassion and grace.

In addition to a balanced give-and-take, healthy communication holds space for both honesty and collaboration. I bundle *honesty* and *collaboration* together under the umbrella of communication because meaningful collaboration stems directly from both parties approaching their bond with the dignity and respect inherent in honest communication. Let's face it, honesty isn't always a person's first choice when it comes to handling troublesome relational dynamics. Being honest about what transpired, how you feel about it, and where you need to take responsibility for exacerbating the issues at hand takes much more energy and willingness to tolerate discomfort than it does to gloss over and avoid the truth. Relationships are collaborative projects built with the consistent input of all involved. If the input is based on fallacy or resistance to the joint creation of the dynamic, it only makes sense that the relationship would edge closer to dysfunction than growth. In *Dare to Lead*, Brené Brown says, "Clear is kind. Unclear is unkind."[2] She hits the nail on the head by identifying the powerful act of service it is when we approach conversations and communications (verbally and nonverbally) with clarity, truth, and honesty. Avoiding the truth does not make it any less true. It simply places a gauzy curtain atop what is real and temporarily obscures it—only for the curtain to later slip off at a wildly inconvenient moment, exposing the uncomfortable truth that had been present all along.

Bottom line: You play an important role in constructing and cultivating collaborative relational dynamics in each of your many relationships. Your honest participation is fundamental to floating that boat. So be truthful with your words, actions, and energetics, and do the work to increase your threshold for receiving the truth from others. Then give, take, listen, and share with consistency and care, and your conscious communication will serve as an impactful tool for elevating your relationship dynamics.

> **How-To Tip**   List different relational areas where you feel your communication is strong. Next, note areas in your relationships where communication feels weak or flimsy. Journal about what missing pieces may cause the communication issue: avoidance of honesty, lack of connection, or judgmental feelings, to name a few.

Tool #2: Curiosity

Curiosity may have killed the cat, but it also saved many a relationship. A curious mindset holds space for more than one thing to be true and for you to be wrong about what you think you know. Adam Grant teaches about *rethinking*,[3] and it applies here. If you believe that the world (and everyone in it) operates from the sole perspective you see through your own eyes and brain, you'll be missing a lot. Every person exists inside of their own spectacular universe where they are the main character and everything/everyone in their life orbits around them—kind of like the sun in our solar system being central to our eight planets (and whatever we're calling Pluto these days). How does it work, then, when two people who both assume they are the center of the solar system come together in a relationship? Not great unless they can both observe the alternate reality and perceptual differences of the other person. Here is where curiosity makes its grand debut from stage left. You don't have to experientially know what it is like to be anyone but yourself (it's not even possible), but it is tremendously valuable to inquire about another person's reality with an open mind and heart. This is how you learn more than your solitary perception alone can teach. Maybe you have had the experience of thinking that you understand something until another person offers a wildly diverse perspective that helpfully fills in the gaps for you. That is the function of curiosity.

An essential aspect of curiosity is wonder, used as both a verb and a noun. *To wonder* (verb) about the perception of another person allows you the type of openness that welcomes new information and perspectives. *I wonder how Aiysha might feel about the restructuring of the company.* Wondering is central to curiosity because it allows for the unknown to be both important and enticing. The noun *wonder* is about feeling a sense of awe and oneness toward something larger than yourself—like the divine construct of a meaningful relationship or the magnificence of a person you are inspired by. *Wow. Aiysha is truly inspirational in her ability to perceive a situation with equanimity.* You can feel a sense of *whoa* (wonder) while marveling at someone's admirable qualities or your profound connection with another. This

greatly impacts your appreciation for another person's existence in your life.

Curiosity is more than a mental process of thinking. It also
imparts a cascade of biological, neurochemical satisfaction by
stimulating your brain's reward system. Let's get scientific for a
sec. First, dopamine courses into your bloodstream when you
activate curiosity and feel motivated to explore, discover, and
seek something new. Simultaneously, an important part of your
brain's memory bank, the *hippocampus*, comes on board to activate long-term learning. When your discoveries prove to be interesting, your brain's pharmacopeia releases natural opiate
endorphins into your system that ultimately bring forth the satisfying pleasure that comes with a rewarding experience. This
pleasure frees up more dopamine, and you again feel motivated
to further explore behaviors that activate feel-good neurochemical rewards.[4]

Be careful not to fall into the trap of thinking that curiosity
ignites only for pleasurable or positive interests. Our brains are
also highly curious about controversial and negative stimuli.
This results in the same neurochemical satisfaction, even when
we cognitively understand that the reward is based on gossip,
false news, petty controversy, or downright wrongness. Consider how you feel when you see an edgy social media post you
can't seem to scroll past. When I create online content that
touches on controversial or taboo topics, they typically get
higher engagement than my tamer, more socially acceptable
posts. This can happen in relationships too if you are unintentional about how far down any particular rabbit hole you allow
your curiosity to lead you. For fruitful relational dynamics, allow your open-mindedness to be used for connection and collaboration rather than for stirring up drama and perpetuating
dysfunction by continually providing fresh meat to argue about.

> **How-To Tip**   Play with the noun and verb forms of "wonder" in the context of one relationship. How well do you *wonder* (verb) about the other person's experience? Have you taken time to appreciate the *wonder* (noun) of their being? Repeat this exercise for each of your closest relationships.

Tool #3: Action

You can talk the talk for only so long before you must walk the walk. Talk and walk, what? Let me explain: Healthy, thriving relationships require action. They demand that you grow, change, pivot, and rebalance your connection as life progresses. Nothing in the world is stagnant forever, perhaps least of all your interpersonal dynamics, so you must be willing to *do* something when updates are required. Think about your smartphone or computer: If you ignore the ping to update programs for long enough, your operating system won't be able to hang with the new technology and requirements for your device. You can talk all day about how you know you need to update your phone (and genuinely intend to) so that you can access exciting new apps and benefit from helpful tools that were previously unavailable . . . but until you actually *do* the update, your device won't progress. Action is key—in technology, in relationships, and in general life. You must regularly update your relationships like you update your devices if you want them to operate at full capacity. Talking about carving out more time, connecting more deeply, and prioritizing each other's needs is a great start, but it won't make any of those things actually happen. Acting in accordance with those values will.

Step one is making your dearest relationships a priority and giving them the time, space, love, and attention they require. You must swim against the tides of the consuming hustle-bustle pace of life and regain presence. Otherwise you won't have time to implement any meaningful changes your relationships require, let alone notice that updates are necessary. When you devote your greatest resource—your attention—to an important person, you can then take their needs seriously (and they yours). By slowing down and leaning in, you will discover large and small relational needs that may have been unmet for longer than you realize. With your attention, you can consciously act in alignment with the relationship's requirements for health and connectivity. You might notice that a certain imbalance has consumed the relationship, like one parent carrying a much heavier a load than the other related to financial earning, social planning, or childcare and household responsibilities. Rather than simply acknowledging the imbalance, you can resolve situations like these by brainstorming and implementing change. Make concrete plans to somehow help the overworked parent and prevent their burnout and resentment. Discuss the social calendar together in detail. Devise short-term and long-term financial solutions that alleviate stress for the relationship.

A common large-scale problem that often comes to light when it's time to take action and make meaningful relationship updates is when a strong bond no longer exists to hold the relationship together. In a situation like this, longtime friends could become aware that their dynamic is solely based on their history without any authentic attraction in the present. With more information and an honest pulse on the relationship's reality, you can discern if the friendship simply needs more effort and care for it to *mend* or if it has run its course and should dwindle to a natural ending—*move on*. This can also happen in professional partnerships when the parties involved discover that their interests have diverged in opposite ways, and it can play out between romantic couples and in families as well.

Gaining awareness of such relationship dynamics is not necessarily good or bad; it's simply honest. Rushing around without attending to the necessary actions for healing relational problems or instigating healthy change toward better alignment does nobody any good. In fact, it can keep a relationship operating from an outdated version for so long that the people involved feel stuck and stifled (nobody's ideal). Certain actions that are geared toward genuine closure and resolution can be profoundly freeing while others focused on deepening and discovery can usher a relationship to new meaningful depths. Whether it ultimately comes to *mending* or *moving on*, always remember that action is key.

> **How-To Tip**   What action have you been avoiding or deprioritizing in a relationship? Close your eyes. Breathe deeply and envision your relationship. Witness yourself from the outside, avoiding the action you know is required. What do you notice? Perhaps you acknowledge hidden motives for your inaction, recognize something that sparks your desire to act, or identify new information you didn't previously notice. Process your visualization in your journal.

Tool #4: Compassion

When it comes to feeling warm fuzzies toward another person, there tends to be some confusion about what compassion actually is. In a cluster of words that are all meant to convey emotional attunement to varying degrees, compassion can often get interchanged with sympathy and empathy. So let's begin with my definitions for each of these words. I will use the context of supporting a friend in the midst of a difficult divorce as an example:

- *Empathy* is your ability to feel what you imagine another person feels. An empathic response to your friend's divorce might be to feel the heartbreak, pain, and outrage within yourself that you imagine your friend must feel—possibly to the extent of feeling overwhelmed. This includes not only emotional pain, anger, and grief but also physical responses such as decreased appetite, lethargy, tearfulness, etc.

- *Compassion* is feeling warmth and openheartedness toward another person without drowning in your perception of their experience. Compassion includes the emotional resonance of empathy but with an added dose of mindfulness that helps you remember that the experience you are witnessing is not happening to you. A compassionate response to your friend might be a caring swell of your heart, feeling emotional softness for her, and potentially offering whatever support you can give without self-abandoning.
- *Sympathy* is a detached experience toward the pain and suffering of another person that acknowledges their hardship as exclusively theirs and does not open your heart to them in any real way. Where empathy says *I feel what you feel* and compassion says, *I witness your experience and honor it with love*, sympathy says, *I feel badly for you from a distance*. A sympathetic response to your friend would be saying that you are sorry to hear about her divorce and then moving along with your day.

Now that you understand the definitions of and distinctions between the cluster of words I call *the warm fuzzies*, let's hone in on what I believe to be the healthiest of the three— compassion. The capacity for compassion in a relationship is like the grease in an engine. Sure, the engine can exist ungreased for a time, but it won't run optimally or have longevity. Eventually, without the protection provided by the grease between metal parts, abrasion, corrosion, and heat will ultimately cause irrevocable damage. This is what happens in a relationship when compassion is absent from cushioning the dynamic. Like an engine, though far more complex, relationships have innumerable nuts and bolts that range from emotional ties to logistical commitments related to finances and carpools and everything in between. If participants maintain the ability to mindfully relate to one another with compassion, the inevitable large and small speedbumps they encounter along the way will be much easier to navigate. Relationships with this orientation can flex and pivot as necessary because of the smoothness compassion provides.

Compassion requires that you must hold emotional generosity for others, meaning that you are generous in your perception and give them the benefit of the doubt when you are unsure about why they behave as they do. Emotional generosity also offers others grace when they make mistakes. If you are willing to see the world through what you imagine your loved one's lens might be, compassion helps you consider why they behaved as they did and what limitations they might be navigating. Your spouse verbally lashed out at you seemingly out of nowhere? Emotional generosity considers that perhaps she is having a bad day or struggling with something internally that you are unaware of. This response is vastly different than thinking to yourself that your wife is a brat, and likely igniting a full-blown argument that leaves you both miserable and sorely lacking compassion for each other.

Although you can still maintain healthy boundaries and balanced dynamics with others when you embody a compassionate presence, emotional generosity allows you to be more flexible and adaptive where necessary, remain unattached to happenings in the experiences of your loved ones that are unrelated to you, and thoughtfully show up with support where you can. It helps you take things less personally and be less resentful because you approach your relationships with a mindset that embraces Dr. Kristin Neff's term *common humanity*.[5] Common humanity acknowledges that we are all flawed human beings doing our best to navigate this wild experience of life, and we all need grace from time to time.

Compassion not only greases the engine of relational connection, but it also deepens your capacity for intimacy. Imagine that you are in a difficult experience for which you need support. Maybe you're even facing the harsh consequences of actions you know lacked integrity. Consider how differently you would feel if you were met with compassion from a loved one than if they approached you with severity and judgment. You would likely feel buoyed by your loved one's compassion, less alone in your pain and frustration, and more motivated to repair your mistake. When you feel witnessed and held with compassion—physically or emotionally—a natural sense of relief ensues. You feel more comfortable being authentic and letting yourself be seen when someone approaches you compassionately because you sense the humanness in them connecting to the humanness in you. They may not be able to solve your problems, or really even help very much in a logistical sense, but their witnessing presence provides comfort because it recognizes your pain without judging it. A singular experience like this certainly fosters more profound connection between two people, and an ongoing relationship dynamic that is regularly infused with compassion is exponentially safer and closer knit than those that lack this magical ingredient.

> **How-To Tip** Call to mind one relationship that would benefit from more compassion from you. Maybe it's a dynamic where you have been slightly disconnected, rigid, or harsh. How can you open a softer heart for this person? Make art about what compassionate connection in this relationship looks like. Perhaps you will draw your two hearts bonded; maybe a rainbow stretches between yourself and them. Then offer your compassion to them in any way you feel called to in real life. Remember, action is essential.

Tool #5: Boundaries:

It is a common misunderstanding that healthy relationships don't require boundaries. Please hear me when I say that all relationships require boundaries, regardless of how intimate and thriving they may be. I would even venture to guess that your strongest relationships are so solid because they are the ones where you feel most comfortable setting and maintaining the boundaries that matter to you. When you are connected to a person who not only respects your boundaries but also accepts and appreciates them, you've got yourself a gem. Conscious relationships that understand the importance of having edges between where one person ends and the other begins have the best chance of remaining strong and nourishing for the long haul. Just imagine how many relational issues could be avoided if all first dates (and first-time friend meetups) began with *Please tell me what your most sacred boundaries are so that I can be sure to honor and protect them.* If only . . .

Think of boundaries as the edges between yourself and other people that define the extent to which you are willing to give and receive physically, emotionally, energetically, and emotionally. The permeability of a boundary is your choice. Boundaries can be fluid and porous for safer relationships and sturdy like steel when you need to protect yourself in unhealthy or abusive dynamics (walls, remember?). Boundaries are not asks you make of others—those are requests. Boundaries explain what you will do when the edges of your comfort, capacity, and willingness are pressed. They require absolutely nothing on the part of anyone but yourself. Requests are asks you make of others that they may or may not choose to accommodate.

- Example of a request: *Please do not call me ten times per day.*
- Example of a boundary: *If you call me ten times per day, I will answer only the calls I am willing and capable of receiving—and some days it may be none.*

Boundaries are flexible shields that can increase and decrease in size and strength depending on what you're working with. In healthy relationships where limits are respected and appreciated, rigidly reinforced maximum-security boundaries are unnecessary. Dynamics that tend to be disrespectful of personal edges or have abusive and dysfunctional patterns likely require much firmer boundaries. When boundaries are repeatedly pummeled, a person might feel the need to reinforce them to the point where they are more like walls than shields. This is something a person's inner system does automatically and unconsciously when it deems itself under unceasing threat. If you notice that your boundary system erects like the Great Wall of China when you are with a certain person, that's valuable information about the unhealthy (potentially unsafe) dynamic at play that you may or may not be consciously aware of. The beauty of your nervous system is that it has the power to protect you from threats you may not perceive as such on the surface—and it does so with or without your mind's consent.

If you feel like someone in your life is placing walls between themselves and you, understand that for some reason—likely a very good one—they feel the need to protect their Self from you. Before you rush to deny this and sling justifications for why I'm wrong to suggest that you could have caused harm, just sit with the possibility for a while. If you are really honest with yourself, you might discover a nugget of truth in your loved one's perception of you as a threat. Deep inquiry about why this may be happening can provide essential repair in a relationship that may be in dire straits because of your actions, words, or behaviors (even if they were unintentional). It might even be the determining factor that helps your relationship *mend* rather than impacting a painful need to *move on*.

Setting healthy boundaries is a journey through three essential gates: honesty, respect, and kindness. Delivering your boundary with these qualities intact does not guarantee an ideal response of understanding and appreciation from the other person (let's face it, people don't like boundaries), but it does mean that you did what you needed to do in the service of your highest good with strong integrity. This work is simpler and more effective if you set your boundary at (or near) the time when a transgression occurs—not weeks, months, or years later. Moving through the three gates is easier if you have not accrued resentment toward the other person for so long that you have no patience left. Once you reach a level of extreme frustration with a relationship, it's difficult to keep yourself from explosive boundary setting where you say what needs to be said, but it comes out laced with venom, aggression, and victimization. Outbursts demanding a boundary can certainly get the job done, but they can also be hurtful—not to mention, boundary setting in a moment of anger tends to feel much less satisfying than setting one with honesty, respect, and kindness.

If someone refuses to honor your boundary, that's on them. Try to steer clear of the sticky trap of thinking that your boundary is valid only if others agree with (or appreciate) it. In emotionally intelligent relationships, members can respect and honor one another's boundaries with maturity (even celebrate them!), but let's face it, maturity isn't always a person's defining quality. You are responsible only for the way you deliver your boundaries, not for how they are received.

When navigating boundary work, many people realize that they have a tendency to collapse their boundaries for reasons like belonging, safety, security, and fitting in. Remember, humans are wired for community and connection, so we will shape-shift and pretzel ourselves into knots if it ensures a stronger chance for us to secure essential connection for our survival. As many people pleasers may admit, this works only until it doesn't. Consistently camouflaging your needs and self-abandoning in an effort to achieve belonging can quickly burn a person out. As you shed your impulse to sacrifice your boundaries, you could come to realize that your tendency to internally collapse doesn't actually accomplish the results you had hoped for. Rather than achieving inclusivity and respect, your weak boundaries likely work against your deep yearning for connection by teaching others to treat you as though your only function is to meet their needs. It is only when you engage relationships from a strong stance of self-worth and strength, with boundaries intact and clearly expressed, that a fruitful dynamic with respect for all involved can unfold and flourish.

How-To Tip   Write free-form without too much thought about any associations you have with the word "boundaries." Do you like or dislike them? Were you taught that boundaries are healthy and helpful or annoying and difficult? Note where these narratives came from. Then write a list identifying your essential boundaries (for most relationships). Include require-ments for connection vs. solitude, the treatment from others you will tolerate, time you are willing to give to certain rela-tionships, etc. Next, consider how well you honor your bound-aries. If you need to align better with your boundaries, do it!

Tool #6: Strong Sense of Self

You have the best chance of building healthy relationships if you begin with a solid sense of who you are and what matters to you. If you are unsure of who your authentic Self is or have endured so much trauma and conditioning at the hands of others that you are unable to discern your own priorities, values, beliefs, and preferences, it is unlikely that you will attract aligned people. Here's why: You build connections that resonate with the state of being you embody most frequently. If you are so consumed with making others happy that you consistently sacrifice your own needs, you will attract relationships that are invested in your self-abandonment for the sake of themselves. If you believe you are unworthy of love and kindness, you will call in connec-tions that reinforce those beliefs by belittling and abusing you. Nothing in either of these examples is aligned with the essential Self of a person who shows up authentically and shines their unique light into the world.

Look, I get it. Life is a battlefield sometimes. We all pick up unhelpful conditioning and wounds along the way that dim our inner light and teach us that self-abandonment is the ticket to gain the security we need for emotional safety. Even so, it is your job as the CEO of your Self to delve deeply inside and heal un-healthy narratives and traumas you may be playing out that pre-vent you from embodied connection to your essential Self. Do you have to live 100 percent anchored in true Self at all times?

No way. Such a thing is not possible (unless you are enlightened). Instead, it is critical to maintain a connection to your true Self that allows you to get lost and deviate during periods of growth and confusion without drifting into the abyss of *I have no idea who I am*. If you discover that you have lost touch with your true Self in a particular relationship, job, situation, or experience, it is much easier to regain contact if you have a grounded sense of where you found true Self before and what it feels like to anchor into the essence of who you are. I know I am embodied in true Self when my nervous system feels calm, I repeatedly get restful nights of sleep, and I feel emotionally available for others. I have certainly drifted into seasons where I suffered from insomnia, felt anxious, and even the thought of deep conversations with others made me sweat, but I found my way home to Self because I recognized the signs that I had drifted. If you are ready for this work, go find my book *The Radiant Life Project: Awaken Your Purpose, Heal Your Past, and Transform Your Future* to initiate next-level transformative healing for your self-confidence, self-worth, and trauma recovery. Once you get the inner work dialed, the relational work becomes a more doable undertaking—trust me, I live this stuff.

When you have a solid sense of who you truly are when no one is looking, when you stop allowing others to dictate who you should be and how you should behave to secure love and belonging, you will forge a clear path that leads toward relationships that align with your authentic Self. You will no longer live under the pressure of barriers and shields that function to keep you small, quiet, and hidden away. Your unique weirdness will thrive when you learn how to accept and embrace it. And with the genuine ownership of the You you truly are, you will attract relationships that jive with that energy. The healthiest relationships are built by people who participate with an acknowledgment that they bring their own special sauce into the mix and that their magic will not be dulled by or in competition with anyone else's. Thriving connections cultivate the congruence of two authentic Selves in a bond between people who appreciate one another and grow together. This is how foundationally strong relationships support and nourish us.

> **How-To Tip**   Collage with magazine cutouts and online images to create a visual depiction of your strong true Self. Find imagery and words that resonate, and paste them together in thoughtful ways that represent your strongest inner core.

It is my sincere hope that the tools in this chapter, and the teachings throughout this book, have planted seeds of inquiry within you that excite and motivate you to cultivate deeply nourishing relationships. As you meander along this complex, sometimes beautiful, sometimes terrifying journey of life, may you attract connections that serve to teach and guide you to the degree of your readiness. And mostly, I hope that you will trust the cadence of this potent inner work—even when it doesn't make rational sense to your well-meaning mind. Let's always remember that we really do need each other. Together we survive. Together we are stronger. Together we thrive. And you are absolutely never alone.

Epilogue

I Hope You Choose You

When we come together collectively, powerful things happen. This is possible in one-on-one relationships and partnerships and also in large groups—even spanning to encompass the collective of our planet. In *IntraConnected*,[1] Dan Siegel wields his magical neurobiological approach to teach the power of MWe (Me + We). Siegel discusses how we are all connected to one another at a scope that extends far beyond each human body, even though we so often feel isolated, separated, and alone. Siegel is not the only poignant researcher to drive home the importance of holding a wide-lens perspective related to the power of relationships. Dacher Keltner also teaches this concept with his research on the science of awe. In his book, Keltner shares a catchy term coined by Emile Durkheim—"collective effervescence"[2]—that highlights the power of collective intention. Durkheim defines collective effervescence as a sense of deep connectedness and oneness in shared events, belief systems, and joint processes experienced by a group of people.

One moving group experience from 1993 was studied over a period of seven weeks when a mass of people set the intention to reduce crime in Washington, DC by meditating together.[3] It started with eight hundred meditators and, through seven weeks, grew to the impressive size of four thousand participants. Before the meditation began, researchers projected that they expected the experience would reduce Washington, DC's crime by 20 percent during the summer, which is traditionally the season with the highest crime rate in the area. When the experiment started, the outcome fulfilled its prediction. Crime dropped each week in accordance with the increase of meditators. Near the end of the experience, when crime had decreased by over 23 percent, the group of meditators was at its largest number. This study is staggering because it challenges the statistical probability that such results would occur naturally or by chance (without group meditation) as being less than two in one billion.

Thanks to studies like these, we now know that group intention and connection can reach far wider and broader than our human minds and modern scientific tools can fully measure. Even without complete understanding of how such phenomena happen, studies like the Washington, DC experience prove that large-scale change is possible when crowds of people gather, and everyday individual relationships can contribute to this movement. If you supercharge your personal connections with the trust and effort necessary to maintain thriving interpersonal bonds, you positively impact the whole by radiating that light into the masses. Your healthy relationships pour into the collective and bring it more love.

If the magnitude of this feels overwhelming, consider conscious conversations as a good place to start—even between You and your Self. Simply begin by initiating an internal conversation about the kind of person you want to be in connection with others and how you choose to show up in congruity with the values you hold dear. Introspection of this kind will emanate your intention outward into direct collaboration with everyone you interface with. When you allow your inner conversation about conscious relational participation to expand beyond yourself and into your friendships, partnerships, work relationships, book club community, and beyond, you do your part to impact radical global change for the betterment of all. This, my friend, is why the ripple effect holds exciting potential to shape and change our groups and families from the inside out.

Another crucial element of building relationships that positively contribute to a conscious collective is learning how to love people where they're at. You get in your own way when you give in to the impulse to fix or change others, thinking you know best about what anyone besides yourself needs. Just pause, breathe, and ask yourself why you are so invested in other people being different than they are. If we can honor our differences rather than force ourselves to conform and shape-shift to meet external standards, demanding this of our connections as well, we might achieve the rainbow of relationships that brings all of our delightful gifts forward to be shared. You can be sure that the four thousand meditators in Washington, DC represented many subgroups of people. They were not a homogenous wash of clones with every component of their beings jiving in tandem. They simply showed up in support of the intention to participate in reducing crime through meditation. Imagine the dynamic power of four thousand perspectives on how to reduce crime. Consider the influential potential of four thousand unique answers, heartfelt hopes, and dreams for a safer city. That is what becomes possible when individuals join together as a collective.

Group meditation is mind-blowing, but what about the day in and day out relational processes that affect each person in their normal lives? This is where your individual strength of intention and attraction come in. If you can be the kind of person you would most like to attract into your orbit, it will be so. Just as collective intention is a powerful force, individual intention is too. If you choose to participate in your circles, groups, neighborhoods, cities, households, and societies with accountability for who you choose to be and where you're placing yourself in your life, you will contribute to a more cohesive humanity by being responsible for your own part.

As you bravely claim your place as a drop in the massive ocean that is humanity, forward and backward through time and space, try to dodge the fallacy of never-enoughness that is so pervasive in modern culture. If you take one thing away from this book, please remember that love is not something to be earned. It is not something you can be worthy or unworthy of. Love is what we all are at our core. It is something we all need and a gift we are all capable of giving and receiving. Love doesn't have to be deserved or discovered, only allowed. Let's agree—here and now—to stop perceiving love as a reward. It exists within and around us, through and beyond us. As the Washington, DC experiment highlights, when we align our minds together toward something meaningful, incredible realities can manifest for the greater good of all.

I'm in. Are you?

Acknowledgments

Just So Grateful

I am overwhelmed by all I have to be grateful for, so I'll start with my household. First my wonderful husband, Danny. Really, it's all possible because of his support and nourishment. Danny taught me what healthy love is, that it exists. He helped me emerge from the sludge. He came into my life like water in a desert, light in the darkness. The gratitude never ends for this wonderful human whom I am privileged to spend my life with. Stemming from Danny and me, I am deeply grateful for our beautiful children, Bridger and Heidi. These two teach me more than anyone else about the layers of love that are possible between souls. Bridger and Heidi: I promise to always be willing to shift, pivot, grow, and change in accordance with life's waves so that we can grow our connection throughout the years. I promise to remember that you are your own people—you belong to yourselves—and it is a privilege to be your mother. I promise to let it be your turn, knowing that I have already lived the years you still get to explore. I will take myself off the table as someone you and your future partners need to fight about and allow you to make your own choices, mistakes, and epiphanies. I promise to love you through all your phases and stages, steadfastly.

Beyond the walls of my home, I owe so much to Suzanne Staszak-Silva, my editor first at Rowman & Littlefield with *The Radiant Life Project* and again at Hopkins Press with *Mend or Move On*. I came from out of the blue to Suzanne as an unknown name, with an unsolicited manuscript, unrepresented by an agent, buried somewhere in the massive stack of book proposals she undoubtedly had to comb through, and Suzanne selected my book for publication—twice! She saw the potential in me and the value in my work. She gave me a shot when I didn't have a million social media followers and I wasn't the author of Oprah's favorite blog. For this, I will be always grateful. Also, thank you to the entire team at Johns Hopkins University Press for partnering with me to bring this important work into the world.

Teachers and guides along the way nudged my growth and expressive process, and I will briefly acknowledge them: Michael Franklin, my graduate school professor and mentor—I appreciate his ongoing belief in me, and I remain awed by the impactful work Mr. Franklin brings to the world. Miyuki Yamamoto, my mentor, teacher, and guiding light from across the world in Japan: The growth she helped me access has profoundly changed my life. I have no clue where I would be without our work, but I know it wouldn't be my current strong, solid baseline. My heart is deeply grateful for the strength, compassion, and insight Miyuki has brought into my life since 2017. Becca, my sister, my best friend: For all the miles we've walked together (literally and figuratively), the moments, decades, and life stages we've shared—my gratitude for our everlasting bond is endless. My mother-in-law and fathers-in-law, Sharon, Scott, and Jerry: I am grateful that they love me like a daughter, especially when I didn't know what healthy parental love was. And my dad: He is real-life proof that people truly can change, grow, and heal despite seemingly insurmountable odds. We were at a devastating *mend or move on* choice point that for a long time seemed like it couldn't be healed, and then he approached me in a healthy way that opened the gates for healing, repair, and love. Dad: Thank you for doing the work so that you could re-integrate with my family. There are so many others who bring incredible light and joy into my life. I believe they know who they are, though I won't list names—friends, family members, colleagues. I am ever appreciative of the reciprocity, trust, truth, and glimmers of magic in these relationships.

Mary Oliver wrote, "Someone I loved once gave me a box full of darkness. It took me years to understand that this, too, was a gift."[1] I know what she means. Though seemingly strange, I am thankful for the members of my family of origin who live at the root of my trauma. As this book shares, my biological family is steeped in deep dysfunction, and several close family members are no longer in my life. Still, I am grateful for the lessons they brought me. I appreciate the opportunities to heal both myself and my lineage. Without shadow there can be no light, so I have to thank these relatives for bringing me the gift of darkness. With gratitude for giving me life so that I can usher this meaningful work into the world, I humbly acknowledge my family of origin's important role in the creation and publication of this work and beyond. I can write only about what I know, and my familial experiences have helped me to both heal myself and teach this important material.

And you, dear reader. Thank you. I have come into clarity that my purpose in this lifetime is to help individuals heal their inner wounds so that they can bring healthier Selves in contribution to the evolving collective. We change and heal this hurting world by first changing and healing ourselves, and that happens only with your participation. By reading this book and integrating its teachings, you move humanity forward by starting with yourself. For that, I acknowledge, thank, and deeply honor you.

Notes

Introduction
1. Oxford Languages, "Word of the Year 2018."
2. Merriam-Webster Dictionary, "Word of the Year 2022."
3. Latifi, "So Many Young People."
4. Latifi, "So Many Young People."
5. Coleman, "A Shift in American Family Values."
6. Schumer Chapman, "What Research Is Telling Us."
7. Mental Health America, "Eliminating Toxic Influences."
8. Mapes, "Toxic Friends?"
9. Schwartz, *No Bad Parts*, 7–9.

Chapter 1
1. Magsamen and Ross, *Your Brain on Art*, ix–xi.
2. Vernon, "Understanding the Butterfly Effect," 130.

Chapter 2
1. Merriam-Webster Dictionary, "Word of the Year 2022."
2. Real, *Us*, 54.
3. "Toxic relationships" was coined by Dr. Lillian Glass: Glass, *Toxic People*, 12.
4. Campbell, *But It's Your Family*.
5. Picoult and Finney Boylan, *Mad Honey*, 342–43.
6. Grayanotoxin poisoning, also known as mad honey disease, results from ingesting certain compounds in specific plants of the Ericaceae family such as *Rhododendron*, *Pieris*, *Agarista*, and *Kalmia* that contain diterpene grayanotoxins. The consumption of such plants, or secondary products made from them like honey, can result in dangerous intoxication. For more information: Jansen et al., "Grayanotoxin Poisoning," 208–15.
7. Picoult and Finney Boylan, *Mad Honey*, 342–43.

Chapter 3
1. Greenberg, "Understanding the Terms of Narcissism."
2. This term is coined by Kate King in *The Radiant Life Project*, integrating authenticity and integrity into one concept: King, *The Radiant Life Project*, 179.
3. Blake, *Comfortably Numb*.

4. Though not written on a specific page, the concept of choosing courage over comfort is explored throughout Brown, *Dare to Lead*.

5. Porges, *Pocket Guide*, 43–48.

6. Schwartz, *No Bad Parts*.

7. Perry and Winfrey, *What Happened to You?*, 132–35.

8. Tawwab, *Drama Free*, 81.

9. Brown, *Braving the Wilderness*, 136.

10. Mate, *The Myth of Normal*.

11. Frederick, "Why Your Brain."

12. Porges. *Pocket Guide*, ix–x.

13. Schwartz. *No Bad Parts*, 7–17.

14. Schwartz, *No Bad Parts*, 98.

15. Perry and Winfrey, *What Happened to You?*, 217–33.

16. Kessler, *The 5 Personality Patterns*, 115–62.

17. Lindsay C Gibson. *Adult Children of Emotionally Immature Parents: How to Heal from Distant, Rejecting, or Self-Involved Parents* (Oakland, CA: New Harbinger Publications, 2015).

18. Siegel, *IntraConnected*.

Chapter 4

1. Brach, "From Reactivity to Rechoosing Love."

2. These categories are informed by Aristotle's writing on ethics. Aristotle et al., *Aristotle's Nicomachean Ethics*.

3. Pascale and Primavera, "Birds of a Feather."

4. Chen. "What CEOs Are Getting Wrong."

Chapter 5

1. Real, *Us*, 37.

Chapter 6

1. Chapman, *The 5 Love Languages*, 37.

2. Nolan, *Interstellar*.

3. Frankl, *Man's Search for Meaning*.

4. Doyle, *Untamed*, 321.

5. Parker, *The Power of Wonder*, 15.

6. Parker, 18.

7. Parker, 15.

8. Parker, 14.

9. Talbot, "What Does Boredom Do to Us?"

10. Wachowski and Wachowski, *The Matrix*.

11. Dr. Lindsay C. Gibson is the author of several books; my favorites on emotionally immature parents are *Adult Children of Emotionally Immature Parents: How to Heal from Distant, Rejecting, or Self-Involved Parents* and *Disentangling from Emotionally Immature People: Avoid Emotional Traps, Stand Up for Your Self, and Transform Your Relationships as an Adult Child of Emotionally Immature Parents*.

12. Gibson, *Adult Children*.

Chapter 7

1. Han, "You Can Only Maintain."
2. Doyle, "The Best Advice."
3. Summer, "Introverts and Leadership."
4. Cain, *Quiet*.

Chapter 8

1. Jung, *Man and His Symbols*.
2. Schwartz, *No Bad Parts*, 98.
3. Eastman. *Are You My Mother?*

Chapter 9

1. Lisitsa, "The Four Horsemen."
2. Porges, *Pocket Guide*, 53–65.
3. Slepian, "A Process Model."
4. Weir, "Exposing the Hidden World."
5. Weir, "Exposing the Hidden World."
6. Lerner, "An Unforgettable Tale."

Chapter 10

1. Vaillant, *Triumphs of Experience*.
2. Vaillant, *Triumphs of Experience*.
3. Barton et al., "The Protective Effects."
4. Siegel, *The Developing Mind*.
5. Real, *Us*.
6. "Wile E. Coyote and the Road Runner."
7. Real. *Us.*
8. Tillich, *The Courage to Be*.
9. Hertz, *The Lonely Century*.
10. Haney, "The Psychological Effects."

Chapter 11

1. Rumi and Barks, *Friends*.
2. Duke, *Quit*, xvii–xxvi.
3. Grant, *Think Again*.
4. Thaler, *Misbehaving*, 203.
5. Campbell, *But It's Your Family*, 124.
6. Tawwab, *Drama Free*.

Chapter 12

1. Francis, *Epigenetics*, 2–8.
2. Real, *Us*, x.

Chapter 13

1. Doell, "Partners' Listening Styles."
2. Brown, *Dare to Lead*, 44–48.
3. Grant, *Think Again*.
4. Parker, *The Power of Wonder*, 41–43.
5. Neff, "The Science of Self-Compassion," 2–3.

Epilogue

1. Siegel, *IntraConnected: Mwe*, 10.
2. Keltner, *Awe*, 99.
3. Hagelin et al., "Effects of Group Practice," 153–201.

Acknowledgments

1. Oliver, *Thirst*.

Bibliography

Aristotle, Robert C. Bartlett, and Susan D. Collins. *Aristotle's Nicomachean Ethics: A New Translation by Robert C. Bartlett and Susan D. Collins.* University of Chicago Press, 2012.

Barton, A. W., A. I. C. Jenkins, Q. Gong, N. C. Sutton, and S. R. Beach. "The Protective Effects of Perceived Gratitude and Expressed Gratitude for Relationship Quality Among African American Couples." *Journal of Social and Personal Relationships* 40, no. 5 (2023): 1622–44. https://doi.org/10.1177/02654075221131288.

Beck, Martha. *The Way of Integrity: Finding the Path to Your True Self.* Penguin Life, 2021.

Blake, Mark. *Comfortably Numb—The Inside Story of Pink Floyd.* Da Capo, 2008.

Brach, Tara, host. "From Reactivity to Rechoosing Love." *Tara Brach* (podcast). April 7, 2022. Accessed on February 6, 2023. 10:04. https://open.spotify.com/episode/129fxkPQtWIhzV5xkVsllk.

Brown, Brené. *Braving the Wilderness: The Quest for True Belonging and the Courage to Stand Alone.* Random House, 2017.

Brown, Brené. *Atlas of the Heart: Mapping Meaningful Connection and the Language of Human Experience.* Harper Collins, 2021.

Brown, Brené. *Dare to Lead: Brave Work. Tough Conversations. Whole Hearts.* Random House, 2018.

Cain, Susan. *Quiet: The Power of Introverts in a World That Can't Stop Talking.* Crown, 2013.

Campbell, Sherrie. *But It's Your Family . . . : Cutting Ties with Toxic Family Members and Loving Yourself in the Aftermath.* Morgan James, 2019

Campbell, Sherrie. *Adult Survivors of Emotionally Abusive Parents: How to Heal, Cultivate Emotional Resilience, and Build the Life and Love You Deserve.* New Harbinger, 2024.

Chapman, Gary. *The 5 Love Languages: The Secret to Love That Lasts*. Northfield, 2015.

Chen, Te-Ping. "What CEOs Are Getting Wrong About the Future of Work—and How to Make It Right." *Wall Street Journal*. February 17, 2023. https://www.wsj.com/articles/what-ceos-are-getting-wrong -about-the-future-of-workand-how-to-make-it-right-8a84e279.

Coleman, Joshua. "A Shift in American Family Values Is Fueling Estrange-ment." *The Atlantic*. January 10, 2021. https://www.theatlantic.com /family/archive/2021/01/why-parents-and-kids-get-estranged/617612.

Doell, Faye. "Partners' Listening Styles and Relationship Satisfaction: Listening to Understand vs. Listening to Respond." Graduate thesis, University of Toronto, 2003.

Doyle, Glennon. *Untamed*. Dial, 2020.

Doyle, Glennon, host. "The Best Advice We've Ever Received." *We Can Do Hard Things with Glennon Doyle* (podcast). July 25, 2024. Accessed on July 27, 2023. https://open.spotify.com/episode/6VmHDknuQEc6f5rM wkndWl.

Duke, Annie. *Quit: The Power of Knowing When to Walk Away*. Portfolio, 2022.

Dunbar, Robin. *Friends: Understanding the Power of our Most Important Relationships*. Little, Brown, 2022.

Eastman, P. D. *Are You My Mother?* Random House Books for Young Readers, 1960.

Francis, Richard C. *Epigenetics: How Environment Shapes our Genes*. W. W. Norton & Company, 2011.

Frankl, Victor E. *Man's Search for Meaning*. Beacon, 2006.

Frederick, Ron. "Why Your Brain Is on the Lookout for Danger." *The Center for Courageous Living*. Accessed July 3, 2024. https://www.cfcliving.com /brain-threat-detector.

Gibson, Lindsay C. *Adult Children of Emotionally Immature Parents: How to Heal from Distant, Rejecting, or Self-Involved Parents*. New Harbinger, 2015.

Glass, Lillian. *Toxic People: 10 Ways of Dealing with People Who Make Your Life Miserable*. Your Total Image, 2016.

Gottman, John. *The Seven Principles of Making Marriage Work: A Practical Guide from the Country's Foremost Relationship Expert.* Harmony, 2015.

Grant, Adam. *Think Again: The Power of Knowing What You Don't Know.* Viking, 2021.

Greenberg, Elinor. "Understanding the Terms of Narcissism." *Psychology Today*, September 2, 2019. https://www.psychologytoday.com/us/blog/understanding-narcissism/201909/understanding-the-terms-narcissism.

Hagelin, J. S., D. W. Orme-Johnson, M. Rainforth, et al. "Effects of Group Practice of the Transcendental Meditation Program on Preventing Violent Crime in Washington, D.C.: Results of the National Demonstration Project, June–July 1993." *D.C. Institute of Science, Technology and Public Policy Technical Report* 94, no. 1 (1994). *Social Indicators Research* 47, no. 2 (1999): 153–201.

Han, Sheon. "You Can Only Maintain So Many Close Friendships." *The Atlantic*, May 20, 2021. https://www.theatlantic.com/family/archive/2021/05/robin-dunbar-explains-circles-friendship-dunbars-number/618931.

Haney, Craig. "The Psychological Effects of Solitary Confinement: A Systematic Critique." *Crime and Justice* (2018): 365–409. https://doi.org/10.1086/696041.

Harris, Dan, host. "372: The Science of Making and Keeping Friends, Robin Dunbar." *Ten Percent Happier with Dan Harris* (podcast). October 2022. Accessed February 19, 2023. https://open.spotify.com/episode/3PToUZGYCY7cKgMlFJqzMh.

Hertz, Noreena. *The Lonely Century: How to Restore Human Connection in a World That's Pulling Apart.* First US ed. Currency, 2021.

Jansen, S. A., I. Kleerekooper, Z. L. Hofman, I. F. Kappen, A. Stary-Weinzinger, and M. A. van der Heyden. "Grayanotoxin Poisoning: 'Mad Honey Disease' and Beyond." *Cardiovascular Toxicology* 12, no. 3 (2012): 208–15. https://doi.org/10.1007/s12012-012-9162-2.

Jung, Carl G. *Man and His Symbols.* Dell, 2012.

Keltner, Dacher. *Awe: The New Science of Everyday Wonder and How It Can Transform Your Life.* Penguin, 2023.

Kessler, Steven. *The 5 Personality Patterns: Your Guide to Understanding Yourself and Others and Developing Emotional Maturity.* Bodhi Tree, 2015.

King, Kate. *The Radiant Life Project: Awaken Your Purpose, Heal Your Past, and Transform Your Future.* Rowman & Littlefield, 2023.

Latifi, Fortesa. "Why So Many Young People Are Cutting Off Their Parents." *Cosmopolitan*, June 22, 2023. https://www.cosmopolitan.com /lifestyle/a44178122/family-estrangement-cut-off-parents.

Lerner, Harriet. "An Unforgettable Tale About Forgiveness." *Psychology Today*, September 11, 2016. https://www.psychologytoday.com/ca/blog /the-dance-connection/201609/unforgettable-tale-about-forgiveness.

Lisitsa, Ellie. "The Four Horsemen: Criticism, Contempt, Defensiveness, and Stonewalling." *The Gottman Institute*, April 23, 2013. https://www.gottman .com/blog/the-four-horsemen-recognizing-criticism-contempt-defensi veness-and-stonewalling.

Magsamen, Susan, and Ivy Ross. *Your Brain on Art: How the Arts Transform Us.* Random House, 2023.

Mapes, Diane. "Toxic Friends? 8 in 10 People Endure Poisonous Pals." *Today*. Last modified August 22, 2011. https://www.today.com/health /toxic-friends-8-10-people-endure-poisonous-pals-1c9413205.

Mate, Gabor. *The Myth of Normal: Trauma, Illness, and Healing in a Toxic Culture.* Avery, 2022.

Mental Health America. "Eliminating Toxic Influences." Accessed April 23, 2024. https://mhanational.org/eliminating-toxic-influences.

Merriam-Webster Dictionary. "Word of the Year 2022." Accessed August 13, 2023. https://www.merriam-webster.com/wordplay/word-of-the-year.

Neff, Kristin. "The Science of Self-Compassion." In *Compassion and Wisdom in Psychotherapy*, edited by C. Germer and R. Siegel, Guilford, 2012. https://self-compassion.org/wp-content/uploads/publications/SC -Germer-Chapter.pdf.

Nolan, Christopher. *Interstellar.* Paramount Pictures, 2014.

Oliver, Mary. *Thirst: Poems.* Boston: Beacon, 2007.

Oxford Languages. "Word of the Year 2018." *Oxford University Press.* Accessed May 18, 2024. https://languages.oup.com/word-of-the-year/2018.

Parker, Monica C. *The Power of Wonder: The Extraordinary Emotion That Will Change the Way You Live, Learn, and Lead.* TarcherPerigee, 2023.

Pascale, Rob, and Lou Primavera. "Birds of a Feather Versus Opposites Attract." *Psychology Today*, July 24, 2017. https://www.psychologytoday .com/us/blog/so-happy-together/201707/birds-feather-versus-opposites -attract.

Perry, Bruce D., and Oprah Winfrey. *What Happened to You? Conversations on Trauma, Resilience, and Healing.* Flatiron, 2021.

Picoult, Jodi, and Jennifer Finney Boylan. *Mad Honey: A Novel.* Ballantine, 2022.

Porges, Stephen W. *The Pocket Guide to the Polyvagal Theory: The Transformative Power of Feeling Safe.* W. W. Norton & Company, 2017.

Real, Terrence. *The New Rules of Marriage: What You Need to Know to Make Love Work.* Ballantine, 2008.

Real, Terrence. *Us: Getting Past You and Me to Build a More Loving Relationship.* Rodale, 2022.

Rumi, Jalal al-Din, and Coleman Barks. *Friends: The Essential Rumi.* Harper San Francisco, 2004.

Schumer Chapman, Fern. "What Research Tells Us About Family Estrangement." *Psychology Today*, February 19, 2024. https://www.psychologytoday .com/us/blog/brothers-sisters-strangers/202402/statistics-that-tell-the -story-of-family-estrangement.

Schwartz, Richard. *No Bad Parts: Healing Trauma & Restoring Wholeness with the Internal Family Systems Model.* Sounds True, 2021.

Siegel, Daniel J. *IntraConnected: Mwe (Me + We) as the Integration of Self, Identity, and Belonging.* W. W. Norton & Company, 2022.

Siegel, Daniel J. *The Developing Mind: How Relationships and the Brain Interact to Shape Who We Are.* Guilford, 2020.

Slepian, Michael L. "A Process Model of Having and Keeping Secrets." *Psychological Review* 129, no. 3 (2022): 542–63. https://doi.org/10.1037 /rev0000282.

Summer, Melissa. "Introverts and Leadership—World Introvert Day." *The Myers-Briggs Company.* Last modified January 2, 2020. https://www

.themyersbriggs.com/en%20-US%20/Connect%20-With%20-Us%20
/Blog%20/2020%20/January%20/World%20-Introvert%20-Day%20
-2020#:~:%20text%20=In%20our%20recent%20MBTI%C2%AE,
around%20%20the%20world%20prefer%20Introversion

Talbot, Margaret. "What Does Boredom Do to Us—and for Us?" *The New Yorker*, August 20, 2020. https://www.newyorker.com/culture/annals-of
-inquiry/what-does-boredom-do-to-us-and-for-us.

Tatkin, Stan. *We Do: Saying Yes to a Relationship of Depth, True Connection, and Enduring Love*. Sounds True, 2018.

Tawwab, Nedra Glover. *Drama Free: A Guide to Managing Unhealthy Family Relationships*. TarcherPerigee, 2023.

Thaler, Richard H. *Misbehaving: The Making of Behavioral Economics*. W. W. Norton & Company, 2015.

Tillich, Paul. *The Courage to Be (The Terry Lectures Series)*. Yale University Press, 2014.

Vaillant, G. E. *Triumphs of Experience: The Men of the Harvard Grant Study*. Belknap Press, 2012.

Vernon, Jamie L. "Understanding the Butterfly Effect." *American Scientist* 105, no. 3. (2017): 130. https://doi.org/10.1511/2017.105.3.130.

Wachowski, Lana, and Lilly Wachowski. *The Matrix*. Warner Bros., 1999.

Weir, K. "Exposing the Hidden World of Secrets." *Monitor on Psychology* 51, no. 6 (September 1, 2020). https://www.apa.org/monitor/2020/09
/hidden-world-secrets.

"Wile E. Coyote and the Road Runner." Wikipedia. Last Modified October 6, 2023. https://en.wikipedia.org/wiki/Wile_E._Coyote_and_the
_Road_Runner.

Index

About the Author

Kate King's clinical experience is sourced from nearly twenty years as a licensed professional counselor and board-certified art therapist. She is also a professional artist, multi-award-winning published author, podcast host, and creative entrepreneur. As the founder and owner of The Radiant Life Project, Kate's mission is to help individuals heal their inner wounds so that they can positively contribute to the evolving collective. King's impressive professional background combined with her personal healing journey lend a depth and quality to her work that are both unique and rare. King's approach has successfully helped countless therapy clients heal trauma, elevate their self-knowledge, gain clarity for authentic relational repair when possible, and courageously end abusive dynamics that show no hope for improvement.

King's work incorporates a dynamic synergy of brain and nervous system science, psychological teachings, spiritual practices, and art therapeutic creative expression to provide a unique and effective strategy for powerful healing and growth—personally and relationally. Her unique approach to deep self-work sparks psycho-emotional repair among her online following, inspirational speaking circuit, and expansive community of past and present clients and retreat participants from around the world.

King is an active member of the American Art Therapy Association, the Colorado Art Therapy Association, and the Art Therapy Credentials Board. She is also an ASIST trained suicide prevention officer and trained in various art therapeutic, psychotherapeutic, and science-informed methodologies including Internal Family Systems therapy, polyvagal theory, somatic experiencing, neuroscience-informed art therapy, mindfulness and meditation, transpersonal counseling psychology, and interpersonal neurobiology. King's expertise in these areas allows her to counsel, teach, write, and speak on various topics from an eclectic perspective that affords expansive applicability of her skill base.

King's four-time first place award-winning book *The Radiant Life Project* was published by Rowman & Littlefield (now Bloomsbury Publishing) in 2023. This psychological self-help book activates creative, therapeutic, scientific, and spiritual elements that contribute to cultivating a deeply healthy, empowered life. This book was included on *CEOWORLD Magazine*'s top five "Soulful Books Every Leader Should Read in 2024" list. Additionally, it was chosen for the "Top 10 Inspirational Books" list by *Aspire* magazine.

King's 2014 book, *The Authentic Mother*, is a creativity-based companion book that offers artistic, scientific, and therapeutic supportive healing tools for new parents on the complex journey of welcoming a child into their lives. She also created the *Ink & Wings Oracle*, a forty-six-card deck comprised entirely of King's artwork that can be used for personal exploration, reflection, and intuitive development.

King has been featured as an expert clinician on more than forty influential podcast shows to share her powerful skillset and teachings about trauma and relationship healing, art therapy, nervous system regulation, epigenetics and ancestral healing, and psychotherapeutic tools for a healthier, more radiant life. Additionally, she co-hosts the popular podcast, "Everyday Epigenetics." King has also written nearly two dozen articles for various magazine publications and was awarded the "Best Of" award for four consecutive years by the business hall of fame in Littleton, Colorado.

King lives with her husband and two children in Morrison, Colorado.

Website: https://theradiantlifeproject.com
Blog: https://theradiantlifeproject.blogspot.com
Podcast: "Everyday Epigenetics: Raw. Real. Relatable." available
    wherever you get your podcasts
Facebook: https://www.facebook.com/TheRadiantLifeProject
    / @theradiantlifeproject

Instagram: https://www.instagram.com/theradiantlifeproject
/ @theradiantlifeproject

YouTube: https://www.youtube.com/channel/UChxGC02H8i
WIReg8X6ADubg / @theradiantlifeproject

TikTok: https://www.tiktok.com/@theradiantlifeproject
/ @theradiantlifeproject

LinkedIn: https://www.linkedin.com/in/theradiantlifeproject
/ @theradiantlifeproject

Amazon Author: https://www.amazon.com/stores/Kate-King
/author/B00N5872SC

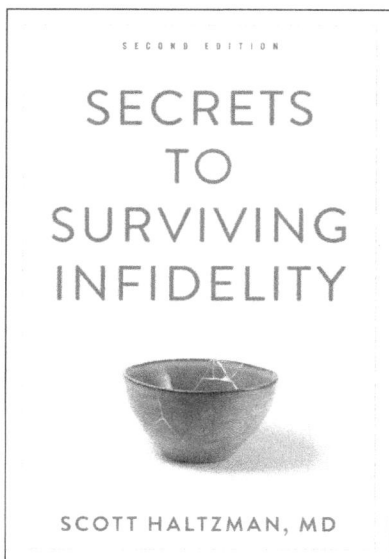

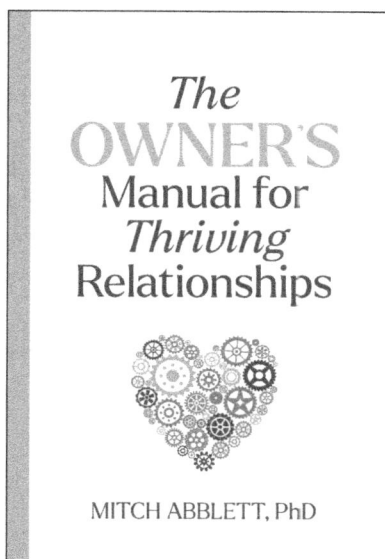

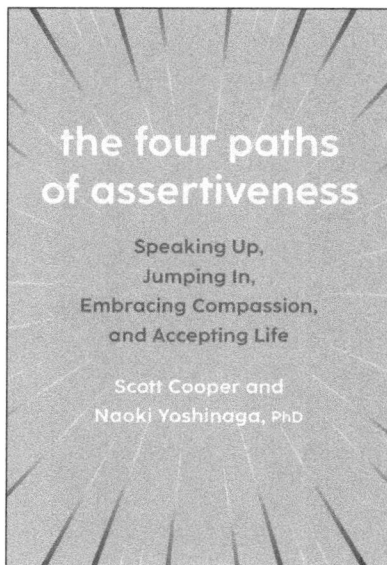

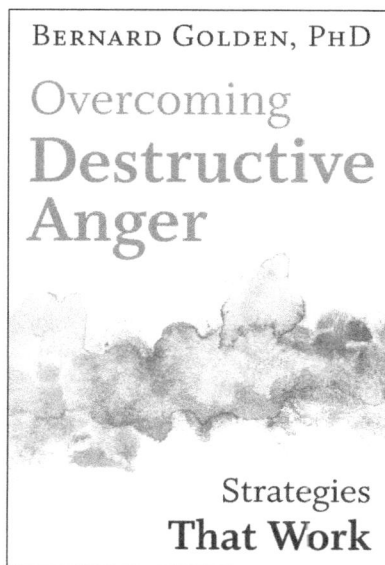